RELAUNCH YOUR VITALITY

ROOT OUT CHRONIC PAIN & FATIGUE TO ENJOY LIFE AGAIN

DR. FELIX LIAO, DDS

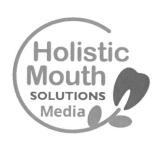

RELAUNCH YOUR VITALITY

ROOT OUT CHRONIC PAIN & FATIGUE TO ENJOY LIFE AGAIN

For excerpts permission, contact info@HolisticMouthSolutions.com

V1.0
ISBN: 979-8-9864268-2-2 (E)
ISBN: 979-8-9864268-3-9 (P)

Cover Design by **Rupa Limbu**

Published by **Holistic Mouth Solutions Media**

Printed in **The United States of America**

Holistic Mouth Solutions Media
7115 Leesburg Pike, Ste 310
Falls Church, VA 22043
800-969-8035
www.HolisticMouthSolutions.com

Disclaimer
The opinions, advice and recommendations in this book are intended for a wide audience of people and are not tailored or specific to individual needs or health conditions. This book is not intended as a substitute for professional medical or dental advice, diagnosis, or treatment. Always seek professional medical advice from your dentist, physician or other qualified healthcare provider with any questions you may have regarding a medical condition. This book is not intended to diagnose, treat, or cure any disease. Significant changes in your health regime should be discussed with your healthcare provider. The authors and publishers of this book make no warranty, representation, or guarantee regarding the advice given in this book, nor do they assume any liability whatsoever arising out of your use of any information or product referenced in this book.

CONTENTS

ENDORSEMENTS

"Dr. Felix Liao's **Six-Foot Tiger, Three-Foot Cage** *changed my life as a person and as a dentist. It pointed me in the new direction of serving as an Airway Mouth Doctor.* **Relaunch Your Vitality** *explains to patients what it is that he is treating and how he does it. I use his 3D Diagnostics method every day in my own tongue-tie and airway practice."*

— **Leslie Haller,** *DMD*

"Dr. Liao has a unique way of explaining the value of wide open airway. Find out how your mouth can bring on your persistent pains and chronic fatigue."

— **Dr. Dawn Ewing,** *RDH, ND, Executive Director*
International Academy of Biological Dentistry & Medicine

"Dr. Felix Liao has been one of the greatest influencers in my dental career. He taught me how to see with new eyes the oral contributions to my patients' systemic health issues. As a result, I have been able to bring on positive changes in my patients that will help them live longer, healthier lives."

— **Dr. Teresa Scott,** *DDS, President*
International Academy of Biological Dentistry & Medicine

"Everyone should learn how deficient jaws affect overall and dental-oral health. AMD Training should have been the first course in dental school."

— **Jeffrey Yelle,** *DDS*
Mountain Wellness Dentistry, Monument, Colorado

"If you want different results, you need to have different perspective. The greatest tragedy for any human being is going through their entire lives believing the only perspective that matters is their own. Be open-minded. Every doctor and dentist owes it to their patients."

— **Dr. Nemie Sirilan,** *DDS*
Oak Tree Dental Center, South Plainfield, NJ

- -

"You don't know what you don't know. Colleagues: it's time to expand your horizon!"

— **Anthony Huang,** *DDS*
Enlightened Dental, Vancouver, British Columbia, Canada

- -

"As a preventive medicine and public health physician, I know how chronic diseases are multi-factorial and inter-dependent. Impaired Mouth Syndrome, as coined by Dr. Felix Liao, connects the mouth to metabolic dysfunction, sleep disorders, chronic pain and fatigue, and more. As these conditions are major burdens on the health care, economic, and work-force systems in America and the world over, the major source is an Impaired Mouth in both structure and usage.

Impaired Mouth Syndrome is a preventable illness. Wellness truly depends on a holistic perspective. I am grateful to know the many connections between the oral cavity and the whole body from reading Dr. Liao's **Relaunch Your Vitality.** *I'm very happy to share this new-found knowledge with my physician and dental colleagues, family and friends alike."*

— **Kavita Rajasekhar,** *MD, MPH*
Preventive Medicine/Public Health physician, NYC

ABOUT THE AUTHOR

Dr. Felix Liao has put the missing mouth back on the healthcare map with his Amazon best-sellers. His books established him as a thought leader in healthcare innovation and as an expert Airway-Centered Mouth Doctor (AMD).

Dr. Felix coined the term "Impaired Mouth Syndrome" in 2017 to highlight the mouth structure's pivotal role in many medical, dental, and mood symptoms. He has shown that correcting impaired mouth can breakthrough many problems resistant to standard treatment. He champions cross-training for healthcare professionals to integrate mind, body, and mouth.

Dr. Felix holds an engineering degree from Brown University, and DDS from Case School of Dental Medicine. He is a past president of International Academy of Biological Dentistry & Medicine (IABMD.org). His continuing education honors include MAGD, ABGD, MIABDM, and Dip. ASBA.

Dr. Felix sees patients two days a week in Falls Church, VA, and spends the rest of his time teaching and mentoring as Director of AMD Training.

Felix came to America from Taiwan at age 16 and has been a U.S. citizen since 1971. His personal interests include classical music, living an organic lifestyle, the outdoors, hiking, swimming, dancing, science, international cuisine and culture, and making healthy food tasty.

FOREWORD I
By *Dr. Steven Lin, DDS*
Functional Dentist & Author of The Dental Diet

If you have ever experienced nagging pain and chronic fatigue, you know the feeling. It's a sense of hopelessness on the way back to "feeling normal".

For millions of people, chronic pain and fatigue is real, palpable, and life-inhibiting reality. If feeling well and energized is something that you don't often experience, know that you're not alone.

Similarly, you wouldn't expect that your dentist's chair is a place for you to better understand the sources of your chronic pain and fatigue.

Neither did I, even though I am a dental clinician. What I have learned is that the sources of chronic pain are a huge societal blind spot. Whenever there is pain, you will find its roots in your teeth and your diet a surprising amount of the time. Let me explain. Eating inflammation-promoting foods, inevitably creates a climate in your body that invites chronic pain. Combining nutritional principles with "root cause dentistry" often causes an improvement in these systemic issues. Only dentists who are trained in functional dentistry addressing mouth alignment and airway can diagnose and treat oral contributions to chronic pain.

This is where Dr. Liao's expertise and his Airway Mouth Doctor Training comes to the forefront. These include your jaw, bite, airway, posture, and pain signals. These are all connected. I've followed Dr. Liao's work for years now and can solemnly attest that he is one of the world's foremost clinicians in helping patients accurately identify and resolve these issues.

As someone with a deep understanding of the principles of functional engineering, I'm always astounded by how Dr Liao turns very complex problems into simple and easy solutions. Impaired Mouth Syndrome, which was coined by Dr. Liao, is a critical piece of the puzzle in every human body that is in pain. Again, in people with pain, the jaw, bite, TMJ, and nervous system are interconnected.

Relaunch Your Vitality is for you if you suffer from chronic pain and fatigue, or if you are a practitioner who sees patients. I cannot thank Dr. Liao enough for publishing this important work that will help so many people, including you and your children.

FOREWORD II
By Dr. Judson Wall, DDS
Director of Dental Solutions, Inc.
Director of Holistic Dental Education Seminars

In *Relaunch Your Vitality,* Dr. Felix Liao calls attention to the foundational law of form and function. If the form of the jaws is narrow and restricted, poor function will CERTAINLY follow. Dr. Felix shows common health troubles can be solved at the source, and it's right under the nose!

"Impaired Mouth Syndrome," as named by Dr. Felix, is a wide range of symptoms arising from a "six-foot tiger" tongue in a "three-foot cage" framed by deficient jaws. This results in a blocked airway and misaligned head and body. Its ripple effects can include: chronic fatigue and pain in head, jaws, neck, back, hips, and jaw joint clicking, popping, limited opening, difficulty falling and staying asleep, teeth grinding, adrenal exhaustion, and more.

Impaired Mouth Syndrome is important to know and treat because it puts the body in an unrelenting state of sympathetic overdrive to survive. It is as if the patient is running from a tiger all day and all night long.

When running from the tiger, the last thing the body wants to do is digest a meal, go to sleep, or become sexually aroused. This leads to poor digestion, acid reflux, gall stones, constipation, osteoporosis, diabetes, hormonal dysregulation, and sexual dysfunction!

An ounce of prevention is worth more than a pound of cure. Your mouth is where disease prevention starts. During my 25 years of practice in holistic dental medicine, I have kept teeth alive by using the principles of good nutrition and supplementation, red/infra-red light, ozone, laser, melatonin, nitric oxide and more.

Quite literally, every vital tooth in your head is as precious as a diamond. Expanding the upper arch rather than extracting teeth can literally change and save lives.

Dentists are in the best position to be the first responders for sleep apnea, a prominent feature of Impaired Mouth Syndrome. Who else can check out your Impaired Mouth twice a year as a source of your fatigue and bodily pain?

A dentist trained in airway can quickly observe if teeth have been extracted for orthodontic purposes. This pinches a branch of the biggest cranial nerves — the trigeminal supplying the mouth and face. Much of the brain is dedicated to keeping the trigeminal nerve happy. When the trigeminal is pinched, the entire body will suffer.

I highly recommend Dr. Felix's concise masterpiece and his principles. His case studies will likely cause you to see the same in yourself or someone you know. The solution involves seeing an "airway mouth doctor," a dentist trained to recognize and treat Impaired Mouth Syndrome.

May you find better health naturally through an unimpaired mouth.

AUTHOR'S NOTE & ACKNOWLEDGEMENTS

Life is misery when you are tired and you have to keep working. Life is hell when chronic pain keeps you from sleeping. This short book shows you how to start rooting out chronic pain and fatigue by recognizing the pivotal role of your mouth in poor sleep, choked airway, and wrong posture.

Energy is the difference between wellness and illness, recovery and collapse, and a warm or cold body. Your mouth provides your body with energy in two ways: usage (eating and drinking) and structure (alignment and breathing). My earlier book *Licensed To Thrive* covered how to eat.

This book connects nagging pain and fatigue with a crucial yet unseen root: a structurally impaired mouth with deficient jaws, crowded teeth, over-sized tongue, tongue-tie, teeth grinding, clicking jaw joints, kinked neck, narrow airway, and more. Until the dots are connected, an Impaired Mouth can start and perpetuate a wide-ranging set of many medical, dental, and mood symptoms that defy treatment, including chronic pain and fatigue.

The problem: As of 2022, the mouth is missing on nearly all doctors' and dentists' radars through holes in their training.

Relaunch Your Vitality tells case stories of pain and fatigue successfully improved without drugs or surgery. The key to solving these cases is the recognition of Impaired Mouth first, followed by multi-prong WholeHealth treatment to restore mind-body-mouth back to working order. The center-piece is an individually-designed palatal expander plus diet and habit change.

Yes, it's now possible to regrow deficient jaws and narrow airway even if you are no longer a teenager. In the new WholeHealth view, all parts of the body are seamlessly connected, and the mouth is huge in whole body health. As long as you have enough sound natural teeth in the right places, you have a good chance of getting out of pain and fatigue naturally.

This book aims to inform you, the owner-operator of your mouth, in a concise manner. To stay short and sweet, I use slides and bullet points; science is kept to bare essentials. Readers seeking more details are referred to my three other full-sized books with bibliographies, which are listed in Resources. You can see videos of patients talking about their own stories through the *Follow Case Progress* link in Resources.

This book provides new awareness and directional possibilities, not individualized medical or dental advice. I will introduce you to a Whole-Health awareness in which the mouth plays a pivotal role, and a new breed of dentist, Airway Mouth Doctor (AMD) and non-dentist Airway Mouth Consultants (AMC). Individual questions are best taken up with your doctor, dentist, or AMD.

For best results, I suggest you read the chapters in the order presented. Before you start reading chapter 1, I invite you to take a survey on Impaired Mouth Syndrome in the very next section.

My deep gratitude goes to all the patients who graciously agreed to share their cases to help advance your awareness, and to all my mentors who have pointed me in the right direction. In particular, I gratefully acknowledge the teachings of Dr. Richard Beistle, Dr. Jay Gerber, Tom Magill, and Dr. G. Dave Singh for his pioneering research in Pneumopedics and Craniofacial Epigenetics.

Great appreciation goes to all the Airway Mouth Doctors: dentists who have taken the training to diagnose and treat Impaired Mouth Syndrome.

I wish to thank Dr. David Gruder for his brilliant coaching, Dr. Leslie Haller and Brooke Goode my editors, Kimberly Whittle for her gracious guidance, BK Suru for expert formatting, Denise Neumann as my better right hand and best sounding board, Aron Plucinski for video storytelling, Jessie Martin as my ever-caring office manager, Chef Franklin for providing *Cook2Thrive* to AMDs and their patients, and Julie Chen for wonderful home cooking and writing space.

Your mouth can be a source of illness and pain, or wellness and vigor. Here's to relaunching your vitality.

Felix Liao, DDS
Falls Church, Virginia USA
January 2023

IMPAIRED MOUTH SYNDROME SCORE
A Self-Survey to Connect Your Symptoms to Your Mouth

Your mouth does far more than eating, drinking, and speaking. Your mouth also supports Alignment, Breathing, Circulation, Digestion, Energy, and Sleep. To do all these jobs well for sustainable health, a fully developed mouth structure is a vital necessity.

What Happens When a Mouth Is Structurally Impaired?

Impaired Mouth Syndrome is a vast set of common medical, dental, mental, and mood symptoms stemming from undersized jaws, crowded teeth, oversized tongue, etc. To see if you have Impaired Mouth Syndrome, fill out this self-survey and discuss with your dentist or a trained Airway Mouth Doctor.

Impaired Mouth Syndrome Score

by Dr. Felix Liao, DDS, Author of *Six-foot Tiger, Three-foot Cage*

Mouth	Score	Body	Score
Snoring, morning dry mouth	0 1	Gasping or choking in sleep	0 1
Teeth grinding, jaw clenching	0 1	Neck, shoulder, or back pain; headaches	0 1
Mouth breathing, chapped lips	0 1	Erectile dysfunction or PMS	0 1
Persistent/wandering dental sensitivity	0 1	High blood pressure, heart disease	0 1
Gum recession and/or redness	0 1	Diabetes type 2, bloating after meals	0 1
Clicking/locking jaw joints, zigzag jaw opening	0 1	Weight gain, pot belly; acid reflux	0 1
Morning headache and/or sore jaws	0 1	Daytime sleepiness, fatigue	0 1
Deep overbite or underbite (weak chin)	0 1	Senile memory, ADD/ADHD	0 1
Frequent cavities or broken/chipped teeth	0 1	Frequent colds, flu, and skin disorders	0 1
Teeth prints on the sides of the tongue	0 1	Obstructive sleep apnea from a sleep test	0 1
Bony outgrowth on palate or inside lower jaw	0 1	Stuffy/runny nose, scratchy/itchy throat	0 1
Sunken lips and reverse smile curve (sad)	0 1	Forward head: ears ahead of shoulders	0 1
History of teeth extractions for braces	0 1	Waking up to urinate more than once	0 1
Bulge under lower jaw, double chin	0 1	Large neck size (M>17, W>15)	0 1
History of lots of dental work + medical symptoms	0 1	Poor digestion and elimination	0 1
Malocclusion (crowded teeth)	0 1	Depression, anxiety, grouchiness	0 1
Total Score		Total Score	

www.HolisticMouthSolutions.com

Figure 1. *"0" means No, while "1" means Yes.*

Impaired Mouth Syndrome (IMS) Score is intended as a survey of mind, body, and mouth symptoms, not as an indicator of severity or predictor of prognosis. The combined score is not as important as the Mouth-Body connections and the resulting solutions.

Experience has shown that many symptoms, whether medical, dental, mental, or emotional, improve when Impaired Mouth is correctly diagnosed and treated. Think of high tide floating all boats. If you have one or more of these symptoms, talk to your dentist or schedule an appointment with an AMD (Airway Mouth Doctor) trained to recognize and solve Impaired Mouth Syndrome.

Why Does Impaired Mouth Syndrome Matter?

Once your structurally impaired mouth is diagnosed, it can be turned from a health liability into an asset by a trained AMD. Benefits based on patient reports include:

- Pain reduced or gone from head-jaws-bite-spine alignment.
- Less tired and anxious from wider airway to breathe better.
- Waking up refreshed and energized from deeper sleep.
- Improved circulation with relaxed arteries, rich oxygenation and nutrients.
- Proper digestion without gut inflammation and toxins clogging your gut, root canals, arteries, and brain.
- Sweet tooth tamed to cut sugar cravings.
- Less depressions, brain fog, PMS, and erectile dysfunction.
- Improve nasal breathing and snoring.
- Bring out your better face: fuller lips and fewer wrinkles around your mouth and eyes without shots or plastic surgery.

Results can vary from fast switch-off of pain in just a few hours or days to gradual improvement month by month, depending on case severity, symptom chronicity, patient compliance, age, total body burdens, and medical complications.

Frequent Signs of Impaired Mouth

Signs are observable "clues at the crime scene." Signs connect the trail of symptoms to a plausible culprit unseen in plain sight — an Impaired Mouth not yet recognized in this case.

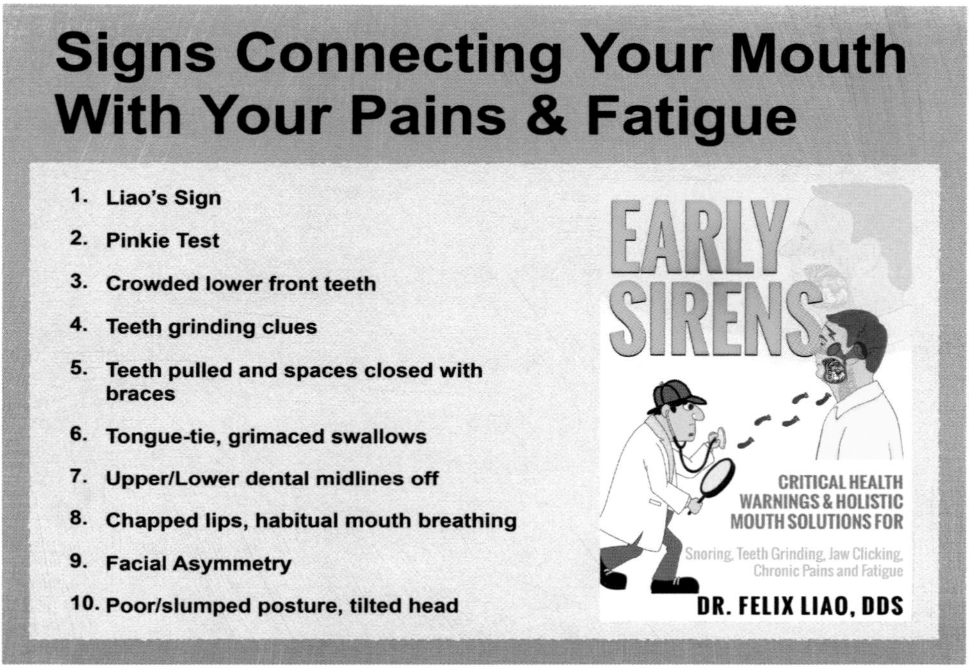

Signs Connecting Your Mouth With Your Pains & Fatigue

1. Liao's Sign
2. Pinkie Test
3. Crowded lower front teeth
4. Teeth grinding clues
5. Teeth pulled and spaces closed with braces
6. Tongue-tie, grimaced swallows
7. Upper/Lower dental midlines off
8. Chapped lips, habitual mouth breathing
9. Facial Asymmetry
10. Poor/slumped posture, tilted head

EARLY SIRENS

CRITICAL HEALTH
WARNINGS & HOLISTIC
MOUTH SOLUTIONS FOR
Snoring, Teeth Grinding, Jaw Clicking,
Chronic Pains and Fatigue

DR. FELIX LIAO, DDS

Figure 2. *Other signs not shown in this section will appear in the chapters ahead.*

Pinky Test

TMJ is short for temporo-mandibular joint in front of your ears. TMJ connects the mandible (lower jaw) and the dental bite to the head and neck. Clues of TMJ dysfunction can include clicking, popping, limited jaw opening, and pain in, around, and beyond your jaw joints. TMJ symptoms are frequent features of Impaired Mouth Syndrome.

Pinky Test is a simple yet reliable test in my experience to assess the presence of an Impaired Mouth:

1. Put your small finger in your ear with the pad facing forward.
2. Open your mouth and close into your back teeth.
3. Test is positive if your jaw joint pushes back against your finger pad in one or both sides.

A positive Pinky Test suggests a higher risk of Impaired Mouth Syndrome, while a negative Pinky Test is a good sign that the mouth is no longer a health liability to airway obstruction, chronic pain, and fatigue.

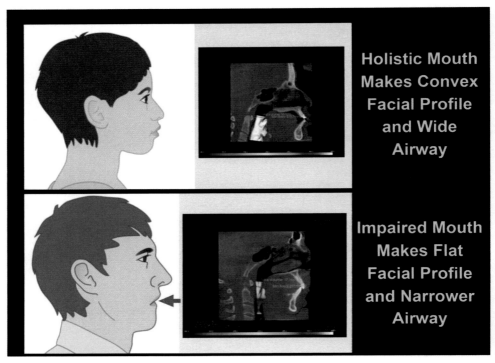

Holistic Mouth Makes Convex Facial Profile and Wide Airway

Impaired Mouth Makes Flat Facial Profile and Narrower Airway

Figure 3. *Left: Facial profile of holistic mouth and impaired mouth.*
Right: Corresponding CT images showing respective airway.

When jaws are undersized or retruded (opposite of protruded), the tongue is driven into the throat to cut down oxygen supply. Figures 3 and 4 show Liao's Sign as a useful surface clue of a structurally impaired mouth.

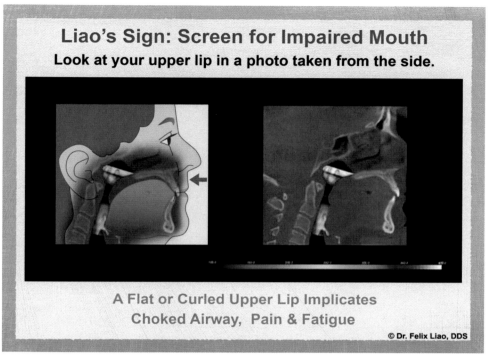

Figure 4. *Color Scale: The airway in white is three times wider than the part in red. The "choke zone" in black part is four times narrower than white.*

A tongue can become "super-sized" from obesity and/or low functioning thyroid (hypothyroidism). This is important for all doctors and patients to recognize. Healthy thyroid function is essential for energy and fighting infection. Figure 5 illustrates a hypothyroid tongue that is not possible to treat with a palatal expander alone.

Figures 6 shows tongue-tie and torus (p. tori). Tori are benign bony out-growths on the lower jaw's inside, on the palate, and sometimes on the cheek side of the jaws. Tori reflect excessive form from excessive function, usually from teeth grinding and jaw clenching to compensate for airway obstruction. See *Early Sirens* in Resources for more oral-facial clues on the downhill slide toward sleep apnea.

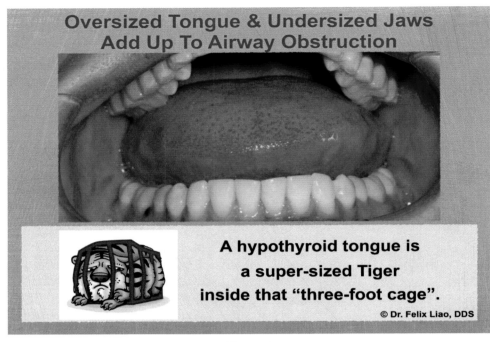

Figure 5

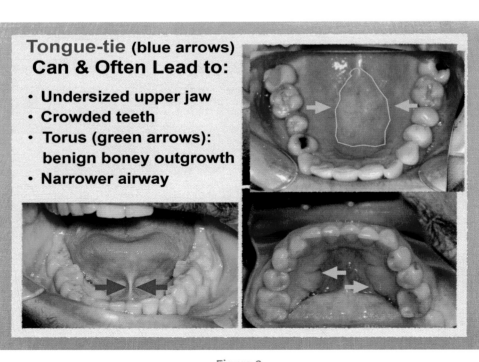

Figure 6

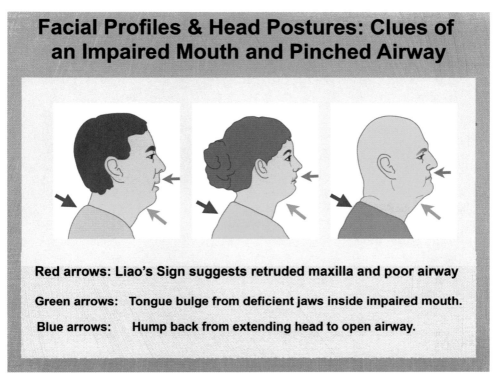

Facial Profiles & Head Postures: Clues of an Impaired Mouth and Pinched Airway

Red arrows: Liao's Sign suggests retruded maxilla and poor airway

Green arrows: Tongue bulge from deficient jaws inside impaired mouth.

Blue arrows: Hump back from extending head to open airway.

Figure 7. Poor head posture from Impaired Mouth contributes to pain and fatigue.

Recognition of these "crime scene" clues by dentists trained as Airway Mouth Doctors (AMD), or non-dentist Airway Mouth Consultants (AMC), or well-informed friends and family can make a life-changing difference, as the case ahead will show.

3D Jaw Diagnostics®

3D Jaw Diagnostics is a trademarked method to assess all three dimensions of the tongue space between the two jaws. It reveals what's off in that *"3-foot cage"*, where, and by how much, as shown in Figure 8.

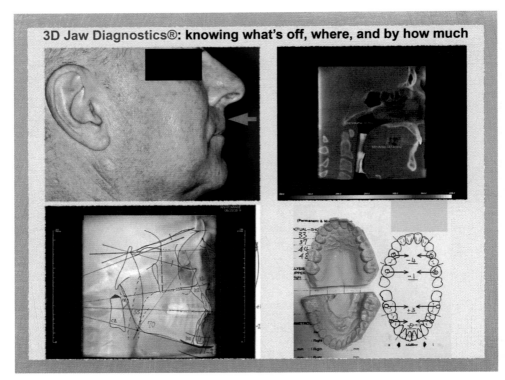

Figure 8. *Top left: Red arrow points to Liao's Sign. Top right: CT image of airway in red-orange zone that's 1/3 the cross section of wide-open (white zone). Bottom left & right: Deficiencies in all three dimensions of both jaws are revealed to guide treatment.*

All treatment outcomes cited in this book came from using Start Thriving Appliance® designed with 3D Jaw Diagnostics® method, plus patient compliance. One pilot's progress reports are shown in Figures 9 and 10.

His WholeHealth treatment plan calls for gradual weight loss starting with better sleep followed by reduced stress eating and increased exercise.

"The oral device does not disrupt my sleep at all, but my CPAP does. Since started using the device, I've started having nightly dreams."

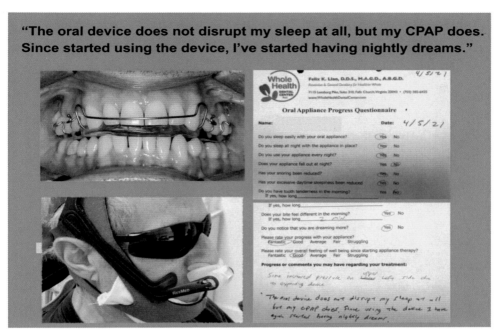

Figure 9. *Dreams occur only in deep sleep.* **CPAP:** *Continuous Positive Airway Pressure device to treat obstructive sleep apnea.*

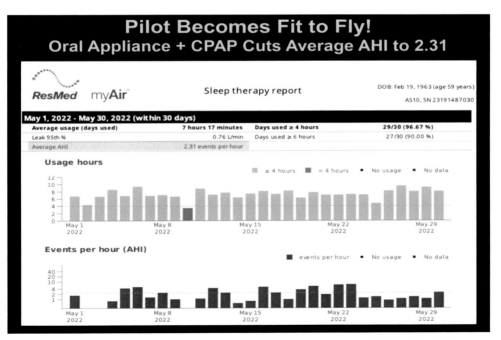

Figure 10. *AHI is a sleep test score. A benchmark for sleep apnea is AHI of 5 or higher. The average AHI for the month is highlighted in gold below the black bar.*

CHAPTER 1
THE MISSING MOUTH
A Gravely Overlooked Source of Your Pain and Fatigue

Chronic pain and fatigue, poor sleep, and "I hate my CPAP" rank among patients' top clinical issues, according to a group of medical, naturopathic, and chiropractic doctors attending one of my lectures. The same with new patients who come to see me.

Your mouth contributes to said top problems and more, including those listed in Impaired Mouth Syndrome Score. An Impaired Mouth can disable you just like a sprained ankle or bad back, except that it won't get better on its own.

Worse yet, hardly any doctors or dentists know that 80–90% of their patients live with symptoms rooted in an Impaired Mouth. And NOT nearly enough doctors are trained to treat it. Let's define a few terms before looking at a dentist's and a physician's case.

Impaired Mouth Syndrome

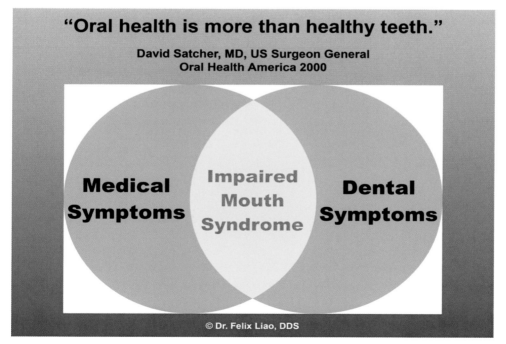

Figure 11. *It's time to widen our viewfinder to see how your mouth drives your health and wellness, or pain and fatigue.*

A syndrome is a collection of related symptoms. I coined Impaired Mouth Syndrome in 2017 to recognize a wide-ranging and predictable set of medical-dental-mental symptoms. Chronic pain and fatigue can arise from an Impaired Mouth. Both can improve when Impaired Mouth is treated.

An Impaired Mouth located at the start of breathing, digestive, and postural systems can negatively impact the whole body. For a detailed list of Impaired Mouth features, see Figure 1 left column, and *Early Sirens* in Resources.

The two jaws form half of the head mounted atop the postural chain. When the jaws are misaligned, pain shows up. When the jaws are undersized, the owner suffers fatigue from a choked airway and poor sleep.

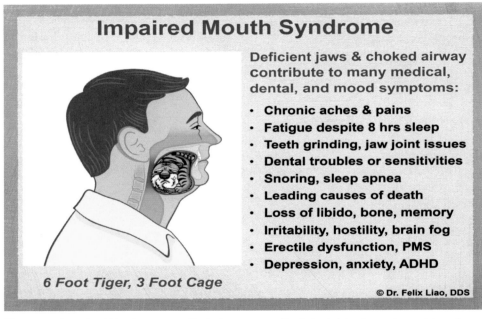

Impaired Mouth Syndrome

Deficient jaws & choked airway contribute to many medical, dental, and mood symptoms:

- **Chronic aches & pains**
- **Fatigue despite 8 hrs sleep**
- **Teeth grinding, jaw joint issues**
- **Dental troubles or sensitivities**
- **Snoring, sleep apnea**
- **Leading causes of death**
- **Loss of libido, bone, memory**
- **Irritability, hostility, brain fog**
- **Erectile dysfunction, PMS**
- **Depression, anxiety, ADHD**

6 Foot Tiger, 3 Foot Cage

© Dr. Felix Liao, DDS

Figure 12. *Impaired Mouth can contribute to many medical, dental, brain, and mood symptoms.*

Each symptom listed in Figure 12 has been improved as reported by patients after starting Impaired Mouth treatment. This means a medical symptoms (be it pain, fatigue, anxiety, depression) or dental symptoms (be it teeth grinding or jaw clicking, or teeth and gums troubles) can be connected to deficient jaws and narrow airway.

Holistic (Unimpaired) Mouth

A Holistic Mouth is structurally fit to support your overall health with Alignment Breathing, Circulation, Digestion, Energy, and Sleep. That requires a fully developed set of jaws, a balanced set of oral-facial muscles forming the lips, the cheeks, the tongue, the throat, and yes, a full complement of teeth. In an unimpaired mouth, Pinky Test (p. 15) will be negative.

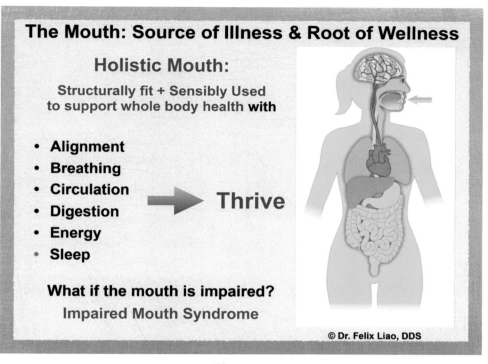

Figure 13

An Airway Mouth Doctor (AMD) is a family dentist with additional training to assess and treat oral contributions to pain and illness in, around, and beyond the mouth. An AMD provides guidance on new ways to regrow jaw bones in adults to uncrowd teeth, align jaws, and widen airway using oral expander appliances, plus necessary diet and lifestyle changes, and teamwork with like-minded health professionals.

WholeHealth is a conceptional model that sees all parts of the body as interconnected, and all systems as seamlessly integrated. We all know the hip bone and thigh bone are connected. In practice, dentists do teeth and doctors mind their own specialty. Thus the mouth is left out of healthcare.

Impaired Mouth is a gravely overlooked source of pain and illness, in my experience. Missing this diagnosis can and does lead to severe suffering, irreparable loss, and high cost from ineffective care. Let's look at the cases of Dr. Sylvia and Dr. R next.

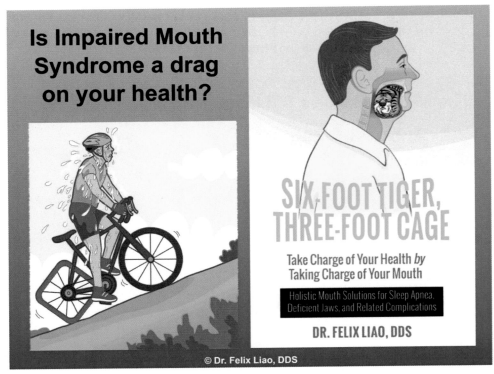

Figure 14

Dentists, Too, Suffer Impaired Mouth Syndrome

Dentists themselves suffer more chronic pain and fatigue than their patients just because of their work posture. Nearly all dentists training to become AMDs admit deficiency in their dental school education to deal with jaw joint (TMJ) pain or teeth grinding.

"I'm living Impaired Mouth Syndrome now!" Dentist Dr. Sylvia reached out before starting her AMD Training: "I have severe chronic TMJ***... I have done lots of chiropractic work, acupuncture, massage for it... even trigger point injections. I also suffer from facial asymmetry, fatigue, typical poor posture of a dentist, restricted airway in my nose and [behind] soft palate, and teeth grinding."

After starting her Impaired Mouth Syndrome treatment, Dr. Sylvia reported her progress using a 0–10 Subjective Units of Distress (SUD) scale[1] to quantify her symptoms, as shown in Figures 15 and 16.

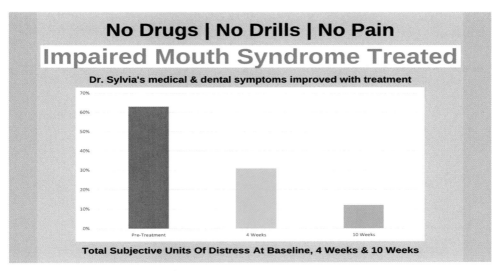

Figure 15. *This bar graph summarizes the bottom row of Figure 16 to reflect Dr. Sylvia's symptom progress.*

Figure 16 shows the details of how Dr. Sylvia's nine symptoms improved 51% in four weeks and 81% in ten weeks. "My TMJ is not clicking any more. I sleep so much better at night!!... I noticed lately that I look healthier and nicer in photos... I am amazed by the ongoing improvement!"

Symptoms	Pre-Treatment	Progress 4 weeks	Progress 10 weeks	Improvement 10 weeks
Jaw Pain	8	2	2	75%
Sleep Quality	8	4	1	88%
Right Hip Clicking	6	1	0	100%
Mouth Breathing	8	6	2	75%
Headaches	6	2	1	83%
Back Pain	4	2	1	75%
Daytime Sleepiness	8	5	1	88%
Brain Fog	5	3	2	60%
Poor Digestion	4	3	1	75%
Total (max 90)	57	28	11	81%

Figure 16

27

Dr. Sylvia's case shows how a correctly prescribed oral appliance plus body work and diet change can do wonders for sleep, headache, fatigue, jaw and back pain. This takes additional training beyond traditional dental schools.

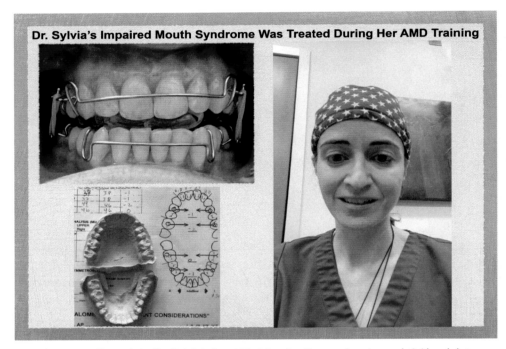

Figure 17. *Upper left: Dr. Sylvia's Start Thriving Appliance gives her painful jaw joints a place to rest and heal. Lower left: Deficient jaw development revealed by model analysis contributed to her pain and fatigue. Right: You can see Dr. Sylvia's video report by clicking the Follow Case Progress link in Resources.*

Not all appliances are created equal. Done right, pain fades in days and weeks, while it may take months to pay off the oxygen debt from fatigue. Recovery time varies depending on symptoms' severity and duration, and each patient's remaining vitality.

Symptoms will improve if a root cause is correctly diagnosed and treated. If your symptoms persist despite standard treatment, Impaired Mouth may be missing in diagnosis and treatment, as the next case shows.

One Physician Needing an AMD

Medical doctors themselves are just as susceptible to Impaired Mouth Syndrome as their patients. Most readily admit the mouth is one big hole in their medical training.

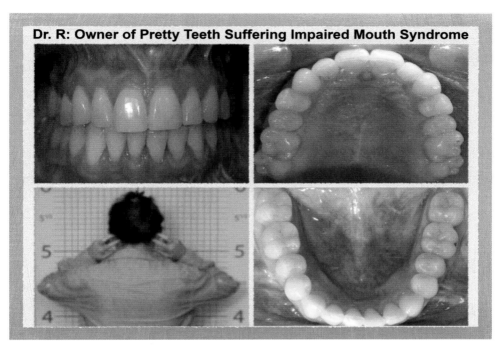

Figure 18. *Images in the slides above and below courtesy of Dr. Max Teja, DDS.*

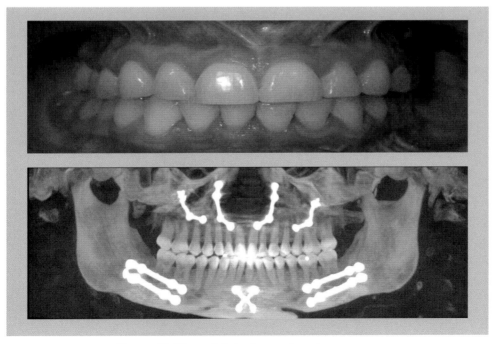

Figure 19. *The metal staples are from jaw surgery.*

Dr. R, a surgeon, had to reduce her workload due to severe jaw pain, migraines, sleep apnea, and brain fog. She agreed to share her case to help others avoid a similar fate.

Dr. R looked exhausted, and her hands were ice cold when I evaluated her. Her health history included multiple medications, plus:

- Full-mouth dental work to cover over teeth-grinding damage.
- Braces twice (a red flag that something had been missed).
- Nasal and jaw surgeries that provided minimal improvement in her sleep and jaw pain — see the hardware shown in the X-ray image in Figure 19.

After connecting her symptoms to her Impaired Mouth, I referred Dr. R to a trained AMD near her to begin treatment using a Start Thriving Appliance® designed using 3D Jaw Diagnostics®. Dr. R's self-reported progress using Subjective Units of Distress is shown in Figure 20. Note the 70% improvement in the lower right corner box, and the diversity of her symptoms her symptoms spans dental, medical, and mood.

Dr. R: 70% Improvement in 4 months

Symptom	Pre-Treatment	Progress	Improvement
Chronic Migraines	10	1	9
Anxiety	8	5	3
Teeth Grinding	10	2	8
Snoring	9	2	7
Neck Pain	9	2	7
Shoulder Pain	9	2	7
Back Pain	8	1	7
Jaw Pain	10	2	8
Daytime Sleepiness	8	3	5
Brain Fog	9	5	4
Poor Digestion	8	5	3
Total (out of 110)	99	30	70%

Figure 20. *With the worst possible score for her 11 symptoms being 110, Dr. R started at 99 and progressed to 30 in four months using only a Start Thriving Appliance.*

Dr. R has since had another jaw surgery to remove all her screws and staples: "I'm so glad it's out. I had immediate relief of pressure behind my left nose and really a sense of release of feeling 'bound down' in the facial skeleton."

All of Dr. R's prior "kitchen sink" treatments missed a critical root cause: her impaired Mouth. Dr. R's Impaired Mouth treatment costs 8% of all her other treatments prior to Impaired Mouth diagnosis. If any of her doctors or dentists had recognized her Impaired Mouth, 92% of her expenses plus nearly all her pain and fatigue could have been saved.

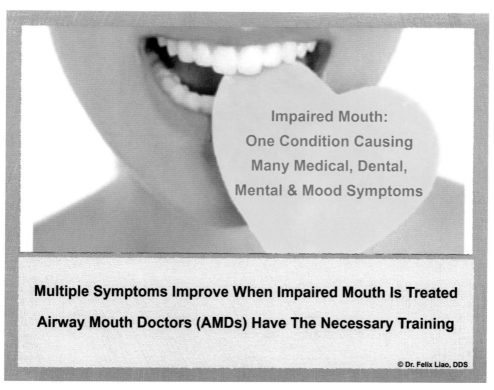

Figure 21

"There's an epidemic of Impaired Mouth Syndrome, yet we received almost zero education in medical school," says Dr. R. "Patients cannot possibly know about Impaired Mouth Syndrome if their doctors don't."

As you can tell from Figures 16 and 20, when Impaired Mouth is accurately treated, all related symptoms improve, be it dental, medical, brain, or mood.

The great news: You are no longer stuck with your Impaired Mouth undermining your health. Better yet, Impaired Mouth treatment involves no shots, no drill, no pain.

Consider trading in your old Impaired Mouth for a new Holistic Mouth if you are tired of putting up with pain and fatigue.

Conclusions:

- An Impaired Mouth can create many symptoms, including poor sleep, fatigue, and pain in, around, and far beyond the mouth.

- Your mouth can be a hugely overlooked source of your pain and fatigue. A trained AMD can help you relaunch your wellness and vitality.

CHAPTER 2

OLD MOUTH, NEW MOUTH
Tracing Bad Back to Bad Bite and Fixing Both

Many chronic pain and fatigue patients have had chiropractics, physical therapy, massage, and more. They'd tell me about the temporary relief and subsequent relapse. Why don't those treatments hold?

The short answer may be an Impaired Mouth lurking undetected. 1,500 swallows a day in an Impaired Mouth will undo daily yoga, chiropractic adjustment, medications or supplements.

Has your Impaired Mouth been overlooked in your chronic pain and fatigue?

Alignment: Why It Matters to Your Pain

The human frame is made of bones, joints, muscles, ligaments, jaws, and yes teeth. This skeletal frame allows us to stand up on two legs against gravity, which never stops pulling us down toward the grave.

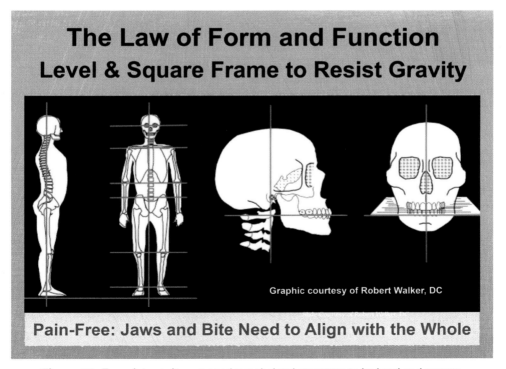

Figure 22. *To resist gravity, we need our skeletal structure to be level and square.*

In anatomy textbooks, a human skeleton is level and square, as in Figure 22. In reality, over 90% of westernized people have malocclusion (bad bite). This has negative effects throughout the postural chain, including pains in the head, jaws, neck, shoulders, back, hips, and more.

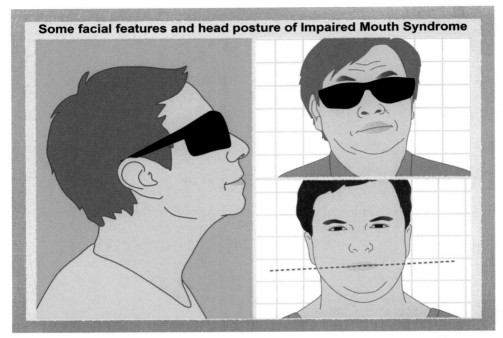

Figure 23. *Left: Forward neck and backward head tilt to compensate for narrow airway. Right: Head tilt leading to pains in head, neck, back, teeth grinding, and jaw joint issues.*

Figure 23 shows postural distortions connected to an Impaired Mouth, while Figure 24 shows slanted jaws and mismatched dental midlines of patient DD. DD came with persistent low-back pain that had resisted every standard and alternative treatment — until his holistic health coach, Michelle D, referred him for Impaired Mouth evaluation.

From the WholeHealth perspective, stopping pain starts with alignment evaluation from head to feet, including bad bite from mismatched jaws. *"I never had a cavity in my life. My dentist and hygienists could never find anything to do,"* said DD at initial interview.

The solution DD needed lies outside the typical dental box of fixing teeth and smiles. Midway through his Impaired Mouth treatment, DD won his club tennis tournament without his usual back and knee braces. You can see DD sharing his case by clicking *Follow Case Progress* in Resources.

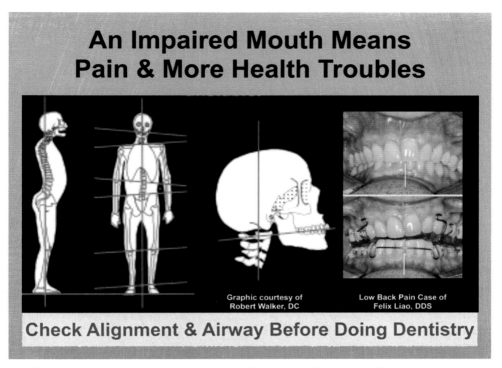

An Impaired Mouth Means Pain & More Health Troubles

Graphic courtesy of
Robert Walker, DC

Low Back Pain Case of
Felix Liao, DDS

Check Alignment & Airway Before Doing Dentistry

Figure 24. Photos on the right show misalignment of DD's Impaired Mouth Structure. Mismatched upper (green) and lower (yellow) midlines are corrected when his oral appliance is inserted, which in turn relieved his intractable low back pain.

DD's case and the next one show how chronic back pain can be rooted in an Impaired Mouth. They also show how a referral to an AMD can be life-changing.

"I never dreamed that my back pain could get better from an oral appliance," said Mr. Miller. His top three symptoms for the fairy godmother to wave away were: (1) a root canal-treated tooth is still sore, (2) nasal congestion, (3) waking up 3–4 times a night from bladder urgency. He also had back and hip pain despite doing yoga, Pilates, and eating quite sensibly.

The more astute reader can tell already that Mr. Miller had a case of Impaired Mouth Syndrome undiagnosed. Let's see why that matters shortly.

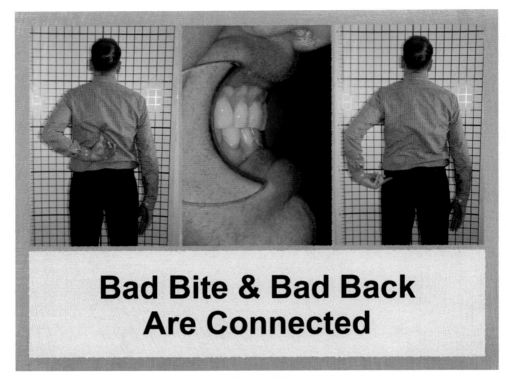

Bad Bite & Bad Back Are Connected

Figure 25

The middle picture in Figure 25 shows Mr. Miller's front teeth angled inward — the result of having four teeth pulled and spaces closed with braces as a teen. This brought on a bad bite that contributed to his lifelong nagging back pain without anyone realizing it. See chapters 4 and 6 for more on the consequences of extraction for braces.

Eating sensibly and exercising regularly can help many health issues, but not pain and fatigue rooted in an Impaired Mouth. Pain from jaw misalignment requires structural correction, most of which can be done non-surgically with an epigenetic oral appliance for adults.

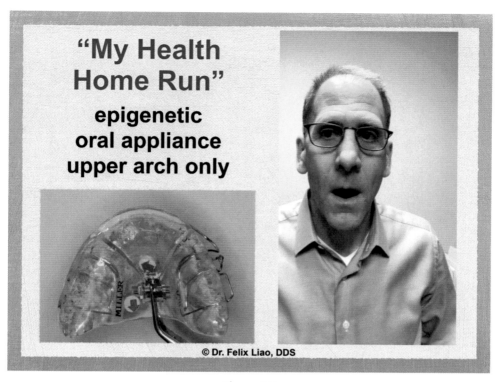

"My Health Home Run"
epigenetic oral appliance upper arch only

© Dr. Felix Liao, DDS

Figure 26

"A mouth piece can make such a difference to disruptive sleep and persistent back pain?!" This is quite a surprise to many patients and doctors. But this is not just any mail-order or store-bought mouth piece. It's a custom-made Start Thriving Appliance® with the following features:

1. Applies epigenetic science to regrow deficient jaws in adults as if they were still teenagers. Epigenetics, says the CDC (Centers for Disease Control), is "the study of how your behaviors and environment can cause changes that affect the way your genes work."

2. Uses 3D Jaw Diagnostics®, a trademarked method to assess the tongue space between the two jaws to determine which of the three-dimensions need(s) correction, as seen in Figure 27.

3. Incorporates a bone-building diet to ensure the patient has all the nutritional building blocks to grow bone. Please see *Licensed To Thrive* chapter 23 in Resources section for more information.

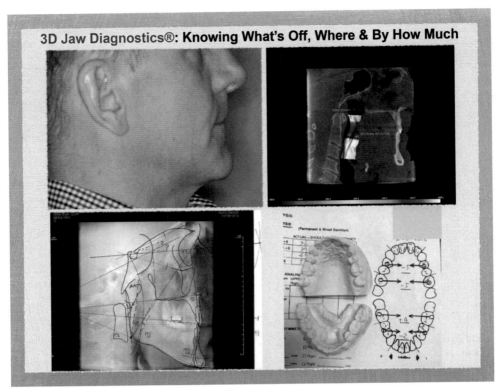

Figure 27. *Lower left: Mr. Miller's maxilla failed to thrive in the forward directions during his growth years. Lower right: Mr. Miller's maxilla (the shoe) is too narrow for his mandible (the foot) to fit into. Both have pain consequences far beyond the teeth and mouth.*

Breakthroughs happen when these individually designed oral appliances are combined with a healthy diet and lifestyle by a compliant patient who follows all instructions and recommendations.

Figure 28 shows Mr. Miller's progress report. You can see Mr. Miller's video comments by clicking *Follow Case Progress* in Resources.

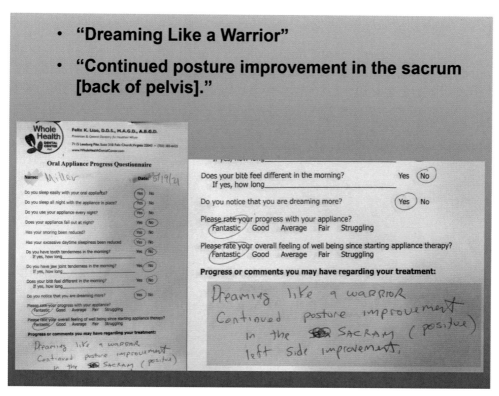

- **"Dreaming Like a Warrior"**

- **"Continued posture improvement in the sacrum [back of pelvis]."**

Figure 28. *Dreaming happens only in deep restorative sleep.*

WholeHealth Integration

A correctly designed Start Thriving Appliance® can treat oral contributions to chronic pain and fatigue. An AMD's treatment plan does not include just a mouth piece, however. It includes referrals for other healthcare professionals to restore whole body health beyond the mouth. Here's Mr. Miller's latest email update:

"My airway and breathing are much more open from my Start Thriving Appliance therapy. My left TMJ has settled down and is holding the new position with wider opening."

Cranio-Sacral Therapy (CST)

Mr. Miller continued, "Even though I don't fully understand how cranial sacral therapy works, it's turning out to be a powerful natural healing method that is helping my body unwind from years of back, neck, hip, and breathing issues mostly due to my narrow palate made smaller by orthodontics with 4 teeth extracted. It has led to:

- My sacrum and hips self-adjusted a couple of days after the first treatment.

- My middle thoracic (chest and mid-back) self-adjusted about a week after my second treatment.

- Another level of tension release beyond my prior spinal adjustments and felt more like a permanent structural change.

Thanks for recommending Mary the cranio-sacral therapist."

To make treatment even more powerful, a trained AMD asks this question: "What else does this patient need besides an oral appliance?" The answer is different for every patient based on an AMD's evaluation and patient's priorities. In Mr. Miller's case, it was cranio-sacral therapy. For more information on CST, see Upledger Institute in Resources.

"It's so wonderful to have more energy!"

Do you routinely feel tired when you wake up? Do you crave sweets and caffeine to make it through your day? Oxygen deficiency from sleeping with an Impaired Mouth night after night will snowball like compound interest into chronic fatigue over time. The next case shows how Impaired Mouth treatment can restore chronic fatigue.

SK came with pain in her left shoulder and lower left ribs that defied chiropractics, yoga, and Thai massage. She also had fatigue with daytime sleepiness for 20 years.

Dentally, SK had years of perfect dental checkups with spotlessly clean teeth and no cavities. She was ready to start treatment after reading both *Six-Foot Tiger, Three-Foot Cage*[2] and *Early Sirens*[3].

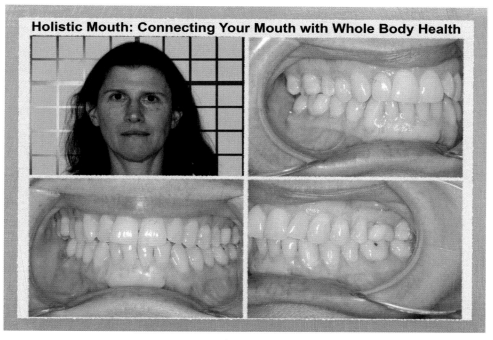

Holistic Mouth: Connecting Your Mouth with Whole Body Health

Figure 29

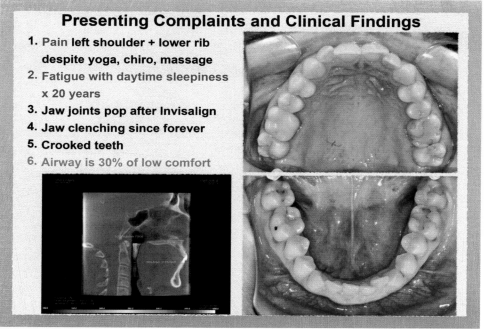

Presenting Complaints and Clinical Findings

1. **Pain left shoulder + lower rib despite yoga, chiro, massage**
2. Fatigue with daytime sleepiness x 20 years
3. **Jaw joints pop after Invisalign**
4. **Jaw clenching since forever**
5. **Crooked teeth**
6. Airway is 30% of low comfort

Figure 30. *Color scale on lower left image showing SK's airway is dangerously narrow.*

Figures 29–31 reveal SK's structurally impaired mouth, while Figures 32 and 33 show her pain areas. SK's airway at its narrowest was 30% of low comfort and prone to sleep apnea. Her jaws were too narrow, so her tongue was forced into her throat.

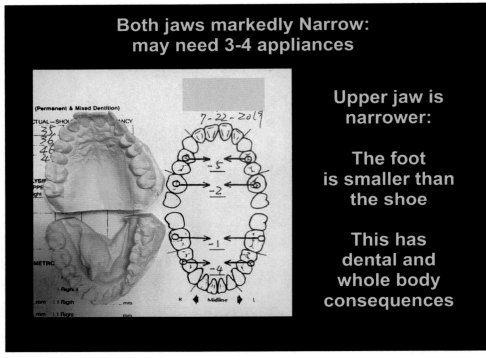

Figure 31

"No cavities" is a good start. But a healthy mouth is more than healthy teeth, as US Surgeon General Dr. David Satcher MD said in 2000 (see Figure 11). Feeling well without pain and fatigue is a much higher bar than clean teeth and white smiles. Yet the answer is right there in the same mouth!

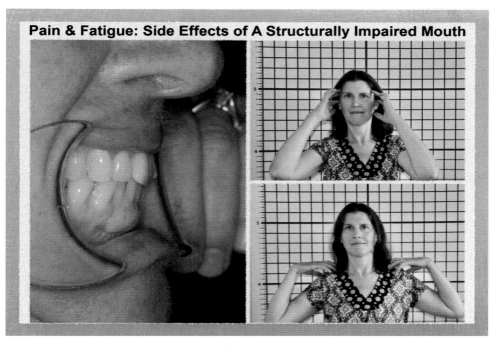

Figure 32

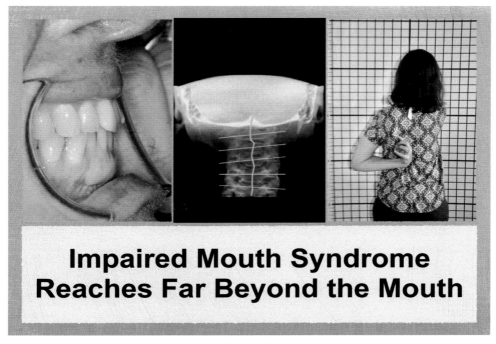

Figure 33

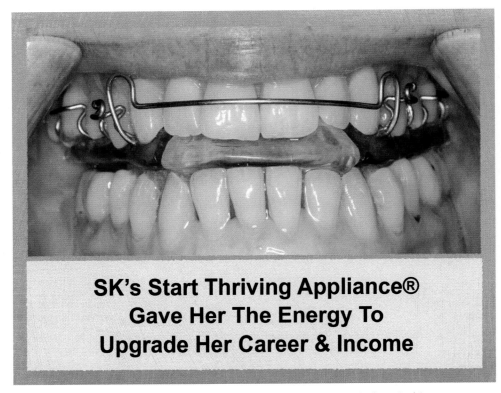

**SK's Start Thriving Appliance®
Gave Her The Energy To
Upgrade Her Career & Income**

Figure 34. *All Start Thriving Appliances are custom designed with each individual's own 3D Jaw Diagnostics, as shown in* **Figure 27.**

Wearing her custom-designed oral Start Thriving Appliance 14–16 hours a day, SK's symptoms lifted within the first two months. Her decades of empty tank were gradually refilled with good sleep along with her already sensible diet and regular exercise.

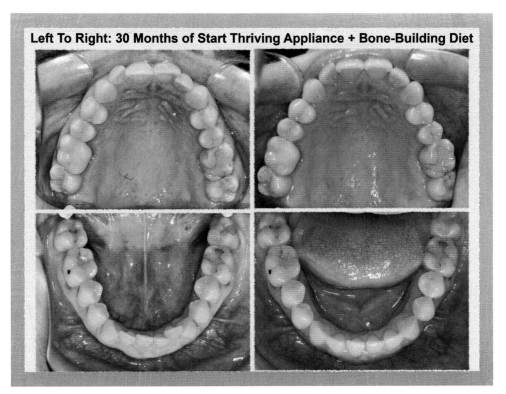

Left To Right: 30 Months of Start Thriving Appliance + Bone-Building Diet

Figure 35. *Upper right and left: Wider palate and less front teeth crowding from Start Thriving Appliance. **Lower right and left:** Lower front teeth straighten without braces.*

Two years after starting treatment, SK reported that she had "much less tooth sensitivity" because "my bite lands evenly and no longer crashes awkwardly." She also became a yoga and Pilates teacher on top of her full-time job. Where did she find her extra energy?

Answer: SK's airway volume increased 64% in 30 months as a result of her jaw growth shown in Figure 36. With her fuller jaw comes wider airway, better sleep, and more energy.

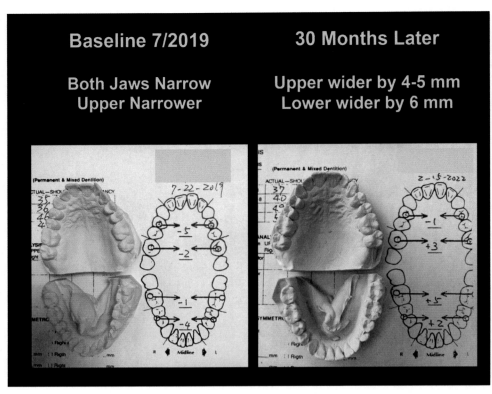

Baseline 7/2019

Both Jaws Narrow
Upper Narrower

30 Months Later

Upper wider by 4-5 mm
Lower wider by 6 mm

Figure 36. *Substantial jaw growth in an adult using Start Thriving Appliance.*

To a skeptical new patient seeking confirmation, SK answered:

1. Process can create gaps but they close on their own; process straightened [teeth].

2. Headaches 99% gone. Used to have monthly migraines.

3. Neck pain continues to improve but I paired it with cranio-sacral therapy at his [Dr Liao's] recommendation and that was the key.

4. Sleep is better. Energy is higher. I even dream now. I now have two careers because I feel so much better.

Also, I had to learn to trust that the healing comes from me... Blessings, SK.

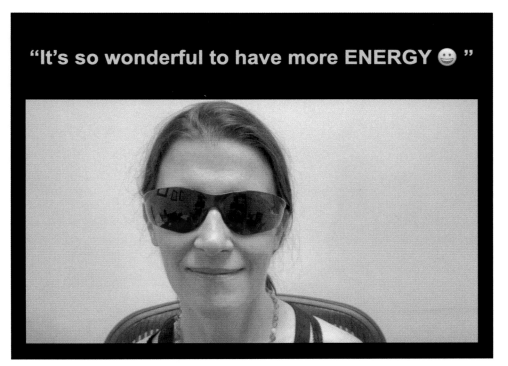

Figure 37. *You can hear SK's video comments by clicking Follow Case Progress in Resources.*

You, too, can relaunch your health and reclaim your energy by trading in your Impaired Mouth for a Holistic Mouth. This is done by seeing a dentist trained as an AMD — see chapters 4 and 6 ahead.

Conclusions:

- If your chronic pain and fatigue persist despite treatment attempts, Impaired Mouth may be lurking undiagnosed.

- Start with Impaired Mouth Syndrome self-survey on page 13. Then discuss with your dentist, or consult an Airway Mouth Doctor trained to diagnose and treat cases shown in this book.

- Adding WholeHealth Integration can powerfully amplify Impaired Mouth treatment. This means a trained AMD may refer you to like-minded healthcare professionals for support in areas beyond a dentist's license.

CHAPTER 3
HIP HIP HOORAY!!!
"Zero pain last night — so grateful!"

Impaired Mouth is routinely a hidden health blocker. Some Impaired Mouths can lead to disabling hip and back pain. The next four slides tell the story of MS's case.

Hip Hip Hooray!!!

MS came complaining of hip pain over the last seven years that limited her walking, poor sleep only in two-hour chunks, overweight, and CPAP intolerance. After her Impaired Mouth was diagnosed, her treatment plan included an upper Start Thriving Appliance and a diet change as the COVID-19 lock down was starting. Her hip replacement surgery had just been canceled by her hospital.

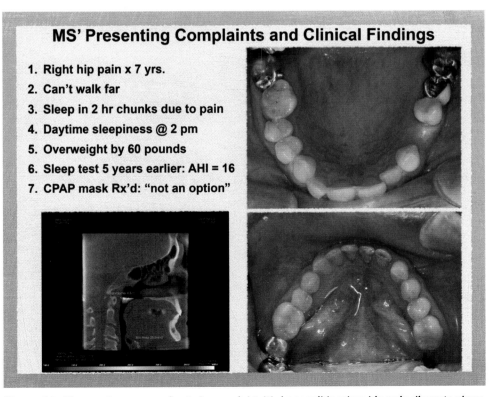

MS' Presenting Complaints and Clinical Findings

1. **Right hip pain x 7 yrs.**
2. **Can't walk far**
3. **Sleep in 2 hr chunks due to pain**
4. **Daytime sleepiness @ 2 pm**
5. **Overweight by 60 pounds**
6. **Sleep test 5 years earlier: AHI = 16**
7. **CPAP mask Rx'd: "not an option"**

Figure 38. *It's easy to say exercise to lose weight. It's impossible when hip pain disrupts sleep.*

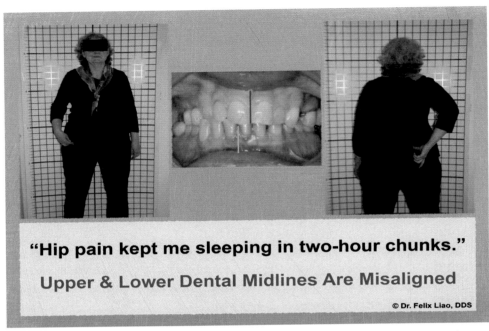

"Hip pain kept me sleeping in two-hour chunks."

Upper & Lower Dental Midlines Are Misaligned

© Dr. Felix Liao, DDS

Figure 39. *Low-back pain can come from upper and lower midlines (blue and orange) off. This is due to cross bite (yellow arrow in the molars) shown in **Figure 40**.*

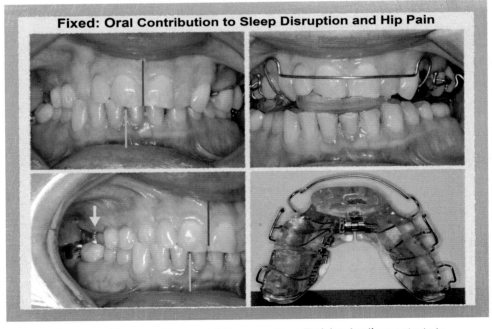

Fixed: Oral Contribution to Sleep Disruption and Hip Pain

Figure 40. **Upper and Lower right images:** *Start Thriving Appliance starts to align midlines and regrow deficient maxilla with cross bite (yellow arrows).*

Five weeks after starting her Start Thriving Appliance, MS sent a text message, shown in Figure 41.

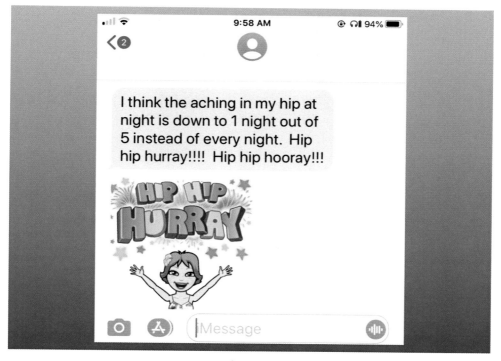

Figure 41

"NO MORE!!!"

One year later, MS emailed: "I can't believe how free I feel, and younger and more playful somehow... You had mentioned that my pre-existing crowns were perpetuating my cross bite. So I followed your advice to replace them with flat temporary crowns that do not engage with the opposing teeth. I can't believe the difference in just 36 hours... I used to have:

- Tight right jaw. NO MORE.
- Droopy left corner of my mouth. NO MORE.
- After standing for more than 15 minutes, I'd feel tired, need to lean on something or to sit down. NO MORE.
- Tenderness in the muscles on the side of my face. NO MORE.

These are all symptoms I have had my whole life (I'm almost 70 years old). NO MORE!!!"

Lessons from MS's case:

A. Impaired Mouth can, and often does, contribute to hip and back pain. MS's and the two cases in chapter 2 all show this connection.

B. Well-done dental work can sometimes perpetuate a bad bite and unintentionally cause pain beyond the mouth in the absence of Whole-Health awareness.

C. Impaired mouth correctly diagnosed and treated can lead to sleeping through the night pain free, plus looking and feeling younger.

D. Age is not a factor as long as sound natural teeth are present.

Whole body health starts with a holistic mouth that can support alignment (to reduce pain without drugs) and airway (to deepen sleep). An AMD can help identify and treat Impaired Mouth's contributions to nagging pain and fatigue. Click *Follow Case Progress* link in Resources to see MS's video comments.

Fixing Pain Needs WholeHealth Teamwork

Gravity never stops, neither does Murphy's Law. Bumps on life's journey will happen, so do small and big hits to your body. Misalignment is the start of chronic pain and fatigue.

Alignment requires WholeHealth collaboration, as shown in Figure 42. The mouth plays a central role in the last four of six items.

Focusing on just one part or specialty will fall short. Instead, teamwork among healthcare professionals through cross-training and cross-referrals can restore WholeHealth.

Features of a Fully Functioning Holistic Mouth include:

1. Both jaws fully developed to provide:
   - enough bone volume for all teeth to line up straight.
   - enough space between the jaws for the tongue to stay in the mouth and not be forced into the throat.

2. Upper jaw is larger than the lower so they fit like a shoe on a foot.

3. Lower jaw is not forced forward, backward, or sideways by an under-sized maxilla to result in positive Pinky Test (p. 13).

4. Head, jaws and spine all in alignment with dental midlines on and no head tilt.

This is not yet taught in standard dental or medical school curriculum as of 2022.

Misalignment Causes	Signs & Symptoms	Expertise Required
Birth Trauma	Facial and palatal asymmetry Postural distortion Face narrower on one side Higher in one eye, ear, mouth corner, shoulder	Osteopathic doctor or cranio-sacral therapist trained or experienced in cranial manipulation (painless light tweaks)
Impact Trauma	Falls and slips while learning to walk or ride a bike Sports injuries Car accidents	Chiropractic doctors Physical Therapists Acupuncturists Myo-Fascial Release
Internal Inflammation	Infections Allergies Diabetes Obesity Rheumatoid Arthritis Various Gut Dysfunctions	Medical physicians Naturopathic doctors Acupuncturists Nutritionists
Airway Obstruction	Chronic pain Fatigue Sleep apnea Anxiety Teeth grinding Depression Wake up tired Brain Fog Cannot fall or stay asleep Slumped posture	Sleep and ENT doctors Pulmonologists Neurologists Cardiologists Endocrinologists Dentists trained as airway-centered mouth doctors
Tongue-tie	Restricted tongue range of motion, grimaced swallow with gurgling sound and goose-necking	Myofunctional therapists Surgical release by ENT physicians or dentists
Misaligned Upper/Lower Jaws	Various medical, dental, mood, and pain symptoms of Impaired Mouth Syndrome	Dentists trained as alignment and airway centered mouth doctors

Figure 42

What other expertise is needed to put my whole body back to working order? This is a useful opening question to ask if pain and fatigue persists despite treatment attempts.

As the cases so far have shown, the mouth is the place to start because it supports sleep, airway, energy production, and alignment against gravity's never-ending pull.

The mouth is not the Whole, however, which is why WholeHealth team-work between AMDs and other healthcare professionals is necessary and desirable for patients.

Airway Mouth Consultants

Airway Mouth Consultants (AMC) are non-dentist healthcare profession-als who have had cross-training in Impaired Mouth Syndrome diagnosis and WholeHealth collaboration. These can include medical, osteopathic, chiropractic and naturopathic doctors, physical therapists and doctors of physical therapy, acupuncturists, nutritionists, myofascial release thera-pists, dental hygienists, dental assistants, dental office managers, and regis-tered nurses, and even experienced patients, with sufficient cross-training.

Cross-Training means knowing enough about WholeHealth to make ap-propriate referrals across all healthcare licenses and specialties. As an AMD, I have learned from nearly all of them to widen my WholeHealth knowledge base to better refer as needed in each case.

Cross-Training also means cross referrals which can make a life-changing difference, as we have seen.

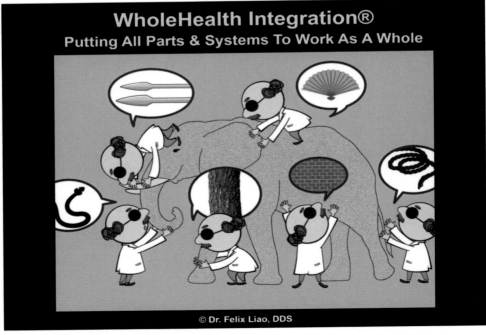

Figure 43. *The mouth is the place to start in cases of chronic pain and fatigue.*

The Need for a New Breed of Dentist

The Earth is no longer flat. It is time for dentists to see beyond the typical dental silo of drilling, filling, whitening, and straightening teeth to recognize Impaired Mouth. It is also time for all non-dentist health professionals to see and screen for Impaired Mouth Syndrome and refer suffering patients.

The WholeHealth era has dawned. The hips and the jaws are indeed connected. Knowing Impaired Mouth's many negative impacts on the whole body creates a new path to more sustainable natural health.

Through no fault of their own, today's dentists and doctors do not have training in Impaired Mouth diagnosis and Holistic Mouth as a solution. Science evolves as time marches on. Nearly all healthcare professionals can use an update on Impaired Mouth Syndrome and collaborate on its treatment. Since chronic pain, fatigue, and insomnia rank among top symptoms driving patients to various doctors, a new breed of dentists trained as Airway Mouth Doctors is sorely needed, as the next chapter will show.

Conclusions:

- Impaired Mouth with its misaligned and deficient jaws is a constant source of chronic pain and fatigue that can eventually handicap your whole body.

- Pain and fatigue are just two of the MANY symptoms of undiagnosed Impaired Mouth Syndrome. Your Airway Mouth Consultant and cross-trained WholeHealth professionals can guide you to root-cause solutions.

- You don't need to be stuck with an Impaired Mouth anymore. It can be painlessly and predictably redeveloped into a higher-functioning mouth to relaunch your vitality with better alignment, airway, and sleep.

CHAPTER 4
TRIPLE WHAMMY
Serious Consequences of Pulling Teeth and Closing Spaces With Braces

Worldwide, crowded teeth is found in "up to 84% of children and adolescents."[4] This issue is not only about appearance but also overall health. Figure 44 shows exceptional crowding in an 11-year-old. Why are her teeth so jumbled? The answer matters to every adult suffering Impaired Mouth Syndrome.

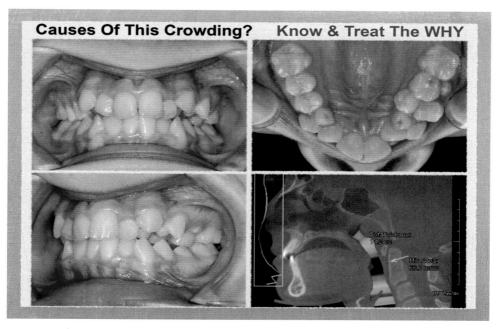

Figure 44. *Impaired Mouth Syndrome in an 11-year-old. Correct diagnosis and treatment can avoid a life of nagging pain and chronic fatigue.*

More importantly, what is the right or the wrong treatment? No matter how bunched-up the teeth may look, pulling new adult teeth to make room for the rest to line up straight misses the origin of dental crowding. The jaw is already too small for all the teeth!

Imagine 16 kids on the sidewalk when a school bus with 12 seats shows up. What's the sensible thing to do? Nearly all 9–13 year-olds I've asked know the right answer — get a bigger bus! The same common sense applies to crowded teeth. Growing a fuller set of jaws is the foundational treatment for your Impaired Mouth Syndrome. This can widen airway, promote sleep, fix fatigue, stop oral contribution to chronic pain, avoid extractions, and still have a straight-teeth smile in all but the outlier cases.

Dental Amputees

Dental amputees are people who had perfectly good adult teeth pulled and spaces closed with braces to straighten the remaining teeth. Straight teeth in such cases come with an aftermath long and wide: flat/sunken midface, smaller jaws for the same tongue, and thus a smaller airway. This results in a worse case of pain and fatigue and a steeper uphill for recovery.

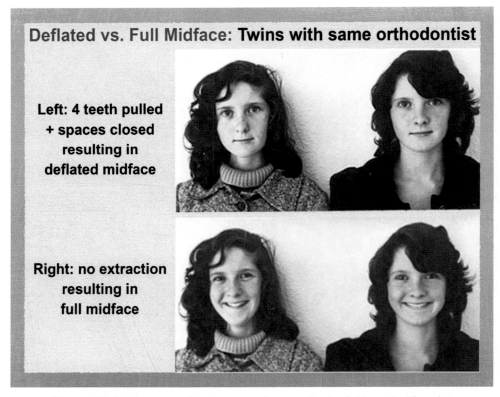

Figure 45. It takes exceptional courage for an orthodontist to make his point regarding the fallout of the extraction approach to treat dental crowding.

Closing the spaces vacated by two or four extracted teeth makes worse an already impaired mouth. Dental amputation cases are among the harder Impaired Mouths to fully recover from because so much bone has been lost. Here's an email typical of dental amputees seeking relief from the aftermath:

"Hello, I am hoping to get information on dentists in my state who help patients with Impaired Mouth syndrome and treat them holistically. In trying to correct a severe overbite, my parents paid for braces, and my orthodontist pulled 4 teeth to correct my bite. I later had my 4 wisdom teeth removed.

Now in my 40's I have trouble breathing while sleeping and wake up exhausted. I am grinding my teeth at night and damaging my enamel and gums. I also need to see my chiropractor often ..."

Time has changed, and non-extraction is a conservative and very viable option because Impaired Mouth can be regrown in adults in the 2020s as long as you have enough natural teeth left in the right places.

Triple Whammy

Crowded teeth come from deficient jaw growth during developmental years, as discussed in *Your Child's Best Face* listed in Resources. This problem has four possible solutions, each with associated health and cost consequences:

A. **Single Whammy:** Do nothing and live with crowded teeth in deficient jaws forming the "3-foot cage" too small for the tongue and suffer the resulting Impaired Mouth Syndrome.

B. **Double Whammy:** Line up crowded teeth with braces but without extracting adult teeth, only to relapse back to some crowding later and still suffer Impaired Mouth Syndrome. The space between the two jaws (3-foot cage) is still too small for the tongue (6-foot tiger).

C. **Triple Whammy:** Pull 2–4 new teeth to straighten the rest and close spaces with braces. This shrinks the jaws and face into a "2-foot cage" with more aggravated symptoms, which in turn costs more to manage and undo.

D. **Grow the jaws to full genetic potential:** Get "a bigger bus with enough seats" to take on all teeth, the tongue, and to unblock airway plus align head-jaws-spine. This can be done by redeveloping an Impaired Mouth into a Holistic Mouth using an epigenetic appliance and bone-building diet to support alignment, breathing, circulation, digestion, energy, and sleep.

For too long, Option C above was accepted as "normal" practice in treating crowded teeth. Having straight teeth was the sole criteria of success. Decades later, dental amputation's health fallouts on the whole body are becoming clear, once we see Impaired Mouth Syndrome.

The good news: Option D is now possible in both kids AND adults, including dental amputees, regardless of age, as long as enough sound natural teeth are present. MW, in her early 40's, in Figure 46 is such a case.

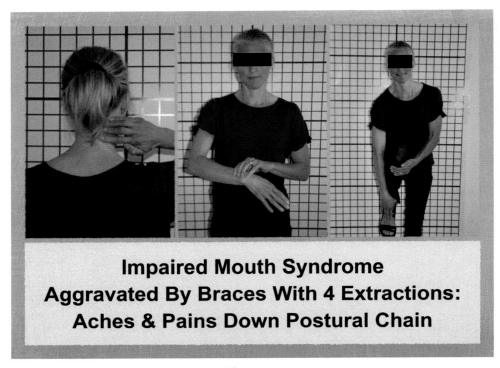

Impaired Mouth Syndrome
Aggravated By Braces With 4 Extractions:
Aches & Pains Down Postural Chain

Figure 46

In Figure 47, the lower left image shows upper dental midline (blue) and lower (red) do not line up. This misalignment is a reliable formula for pain that keeps coming back. In all three images, teeth grinding's destructions are evident in the flattened chewing surfaces in back teeth and worn-down edges of front teeth. The yellow arrows in the right images point to one pair of premolars instead of two in each jaw. Such an impaired mouth structure is a recipe for pain, fatigue, and further dental destruction.

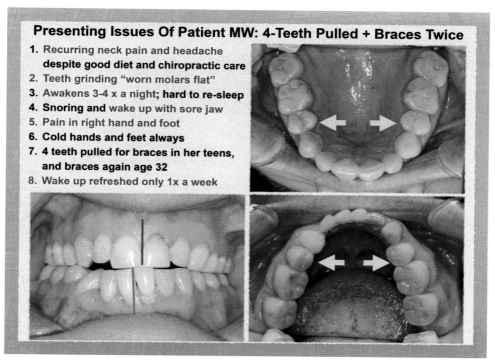

Presenting Issues Of Patient MW: 4-Teeth Pulled + Braces Twice

1. Recurring neck pain and headache despite good diet and chiropractic care
2. Teeth grinding "worn molars flat"
3. Awakens 3-4 x a night; **hard to re-sleep**
4. **Snoring** and wake up with sore jaw
5. Pain in right hand and foot
6. **Cold hands and feet always**
7. **4 teeth pulled for braces in her teens,** and braces again age 32
8. Wake up refreshed only 1x a week

Figure 47. *Impaired Mouth Syndrome is typically magnified in dental amputation cases.*

MW was a compliant patient who carried out all the WholeHealth recommendations on body work and diet change. Her recovery came haltingly because of decades of oxygen and sleep deficit. One year later, MW came in smiling and declared "No migraine in the past eight weeks!" And we elbow-bumped each other.

Extracting infected teeth causing horrible pain is necessary firefighting rescue. But extracting virgin natural teeth just to straighten the remaining ones? No way. Not for my grandchildren. If top health and best face come from fully grown jaws, why would I choose or recommend dental amputation?

Every tooth is entitled its plot of jaw bone in God's plan. Once extracted, teeth cannot be put back. Pain, fatigue, and a worse case of Impaired Mouth Syndrome follow in due course. Undoing this aggravated type of Impaired Mouth is more costly to the patient and challenging to the mouth doctor in terms of treatment time and expertise.

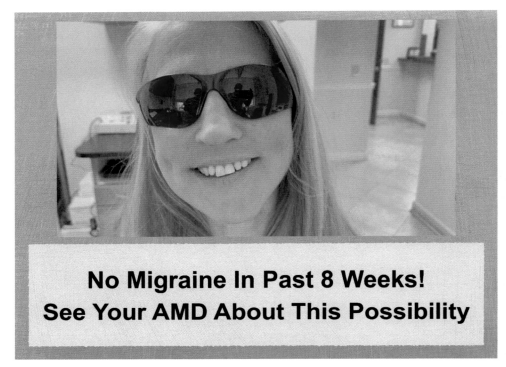

No Migraine In Past 8 Weeks!
See Your AMD About This Possibility

Figure 48. *You can hear MW's comments by clicking **Follow Case Progress** link in Resources.*

Straight Teeth, Miserable Owner: The Case of GS

"I'm unable to breathe fully EVER... not being able to breathe is like a slow torturous death," GS emailed from another continent, after reading *Six-Foot Tiger, Three-Foot Cage.*

"It has helped me to clarify my prolonged pain and frustrations that have led to almost killing myself repeatedly... So I'm writing to you for help and insight into what to do to address this hugely painful, limiting, restricting and infuriating mind and body damage and the suffering I have felt deeply just from jaw, mouth, tongue, throat, nasal and audial issues that were exponentially worsened."

GS agreed to share her case to help educate others to avoid a similar fate.

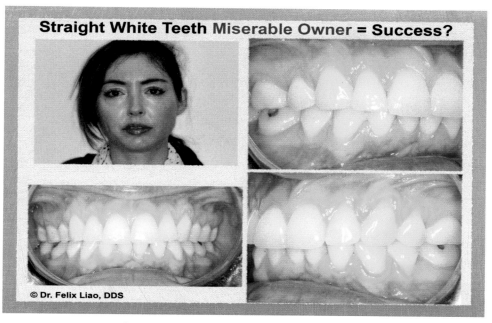

Figure 49. *Above: GS's appearance dentally and facially. Images courtesy of her family dentist.*

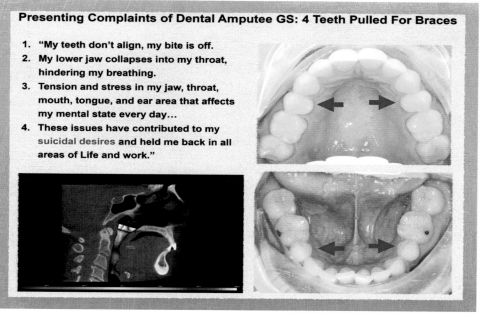

Figure 50. **Lower left:** *Black and red on color scale means GS's airway is 20% of the wide-open blue and white end.* **Right:** *Blue arrows point to one pair of premolars in each jaw instead of two, which means smaller jaws and airway.*

From a conventional view, GS's braces were a cosmetic success. From the WholeHealth perspective, her treatment failed a basic standard: Do no harm.

Mouth	Score	Body	Score
Snoring, morning dry mouth	0 1	Gasping or choking in sleep	0 1
Teeth grinding, jaw	0 1	Neck, shoulder, or back pain; headaches	0 1
Mouth breathing, chapped lips	0 1	Erectile dysfunction or PMS	0 1
Persistent/wandering dental sensitivity	0 1	High blood pressure, heart disease	0 1
Gum recession and/or redness	0 1	Diabetes type 2, bloating after meals	0 1
Clicking/locking jaw joints, zigzag jaw opening	0 1	Weight gain, pot belly; acid reflux	0 1
Morning headache and/or sore jaws	0 1	Daytime sleepiness, fatigue	0 1
Deep overbite or underbite (weak chin)	0 1	Senile memory, ADD/ADHD	0 1
Frequent cavities or broken/chipped teeth	0 1	Frequent colds, flu, and skin disorders	0 1
Teeth prints on the sides of the tongue	0 1	Obstructive sleep apnea from a sleep test	0 1
Bony outgrowth on palate or inside lower jaw	0 1	Stuffy/runny nose, scratchy/itchy throat	0 1
Sunken lips and reverse smile curve (sad)	0 1	Forward head: ears ahead of shoulders	0 1
History of teeth extractions for braces	0 1	Waking up to urinate more than once	0 1
Bulge under lower jaw, double chin	0 1	Large neck size (M>17, W>15)	0 1
History of lots of dental work + medical symptoms	0 1	Poor digestion and elimination	0 1
Malocclusion (crowded teeth)	0 1	Depression, anxiety, grouchiness	0 1

Figure 51. "0" under the Score column means No, while "1" means Yes. GS checked every box except one under the Mouth and two under the Body column.

Figure 51 is the aftermath of GS's dental amputation and Impaired Mouth Syndrome undiagnosed. Missing this diagnosis perpetuated her pain and hopelessness for decades. My heart wept as I read on:

"I have suffered all this pain... since the removal, against my wishes and needs of 8 healthy teeth, starting age 15 when 4 perfectly healthy teeth were removed to 'create space for crooked and overcrowded teeth' ... [which] has led to extremely physically painful and mentally devastating and draining jaw issues, that cause me suffering ALL THE TIME."

With the help of her smart and kind local dentist adopting an AMD's treatment plan, GS started her recovery. In four weeks, GS's symptoms improved 25%, and 67% in seven months, as Figure 52 shows.

GS Symptoms	Before Treatment	Progress Week 4	Progress Week 10	Progress Week 28	Gains To Date
Jaw Pain	10	5	4	0	10
Sleep Disruption	10	5	3	4	6
Snoring	10	6	5	3	7
Neck Pain	8	5	5	3	5
Daytime Sleepiness	6	4	4	3	3
Brain Fog	9	7	6	5	4
Poor Digestion	10	8	5	3	7
Total (70 max)	63	43	32	21	67%

Figure 52. Note all symptoms improve from left to right, whether medical, dental, or mental-emotional. In particular, GS's jaw pain dropped to 0 as reflected in passing the 3-finger test in Figure 53.

As a result, GS is starting to have vivid dreams signaling deeper sleep, and a touch of baby pink is starting to show on her cheeks. Best of all, GS has pulled back from the brink of suicide by finding her purpose in life.

Straight White Teeth: With Health vs. Not

In the quest for straight teeth, the root cause of dental crowding is often missed: stunted jaw growth. Dental amputation imposes a smaller space between the two jaws on the same size tongue, which is then forced down the throat to choke the airway. If tongue-reduction surgery is unthinkable, then why is pulling irreplaceable teeth acceptable?

To be clear, braces have their place in straightening crooked teeth. From my experience helping dental amputees, I am advocating for 100% safeguarding of everyone's airway first and always.

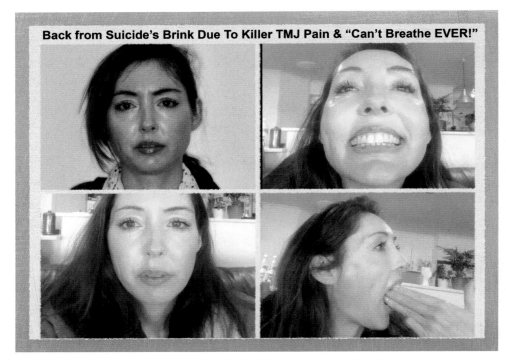

Back from Suicide's Brink Due To Killer TMJ Pain & "Can't Breathe EVER!"

Figure 53. *GS's progress in facial appearance and jaw function after 10 months' of Start Thriving Appliance® + Bone Building Diet.*

The case of GS shows how severe the complications of dental amputation can be. While most dental amputees do not end up contemplating suicide, the suffering from the aggravated Impaired Mouth Syndrome is real. So are the extra medical, dental, mental-emotional, and life quality costs.

Do This Before Moving or Extracting Sound Teeth

By age 16 in most girls and 18 in most boys, 16 adult teeth will be coming into each jaw in place of 10 baby teeth. Sufficient jaw growth, especially in the maxilla, is the key to avoiding crowded teeth and the risk of wrong treatment.

In building a house, the sensible sequence is to lay a foundation, erect the walls level and square first. Then finish the rooms and move the furniture in. Not the other way around.

In the mouth, orthopedic (bone to bone) foundation should be assessed and developed ahead of orthodontic (teeth to teeth) finish. Failing this order of Phase I Orthopedics before Phase II Orthodontics can have serious health and financial consequences in many cases.

The Great News

In the 2020's, it is now possible to regrow deficient jaws, even in dental amputation cases, as long as you have sound teeth remaining in the right places, as we shall see in chapter 6.

Sound natural teeth are vital assets in this new solution. Readers interested in keeping natural teeth sound and safe are referred to Foreword I & II by Dr. Lin and Dr. Wall to see how holistic preventive dentistry is done by leading-edge dentists.

To catch Impaired Mouth Syndrome early and treat it without dental amputations, see *Your Child's Best Face: How To Nurture Top Health & Natural Glow* in Resources.

Conclusions:

- Every tooth in both jaws matters materially to full-sized jaws and wide airway to avoid oral contributions to chronic pain and fatigue.

- Impaired Mouth in adults comes from not recognizing deficient jaws that failed to thrive during growth years.

- Reducing jaw size by extracting teeth and closing the spaces with braces can fuel pain and fatigue that resists treatment and meaningful relief until Impaired Mouth is diagnosed and treated.

CHAPTER 5
EAT TO THRIVE
Your Sweet Tooth, Innate Immunity, and Snoring

Eating healthier contributes to feeling and looking better. Sugar excess leads to not only dental cavities, but also heart disease, diabetes, obesity, painful inflammation, and wrinkles around the mouth and on the face. For more scientific evidence of the dark side of sugar, see chapter 7 in *Licensed To Thrive* in Resources.

Longevity is associated with cutting back on sugar. Longest-lived people in <u>Blue Zones</u>[5] around the world eat a diet of low sugar, low dairy, little meat, and lots of beans and greens, unlike the typical American diet.

Hand-to-Mouth predominates the human brain, as Figure 54 shows. Beware of this neurological pattern the next time your sweet tooth whines. Know that sugar is both disabling and addicting. Let's take a quick look at three nutritional research conclusions that can impact your natural health and immunity.

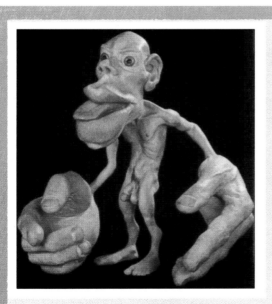

Mouth and Hands Are Big In Your Brain

Homunculus:

number of neurons devoted to each body part

Penfield, W. and Rasmussen, T. (1950) The Cerebral Cortex of Man: A Clinical Study of Localization of Function. Macmillan, Oxford.

Figure 54

"Intense Sweetness Surpasses Cocaine Rewards"

Eating sugar can paralyze your immune cells that kill bacteria for up to five hours. Yes, that was reported in a <u>1973 study</u>[6] by Sanchez et al, plus it took fasting 36–60 hours to restore that immune power.

When trying to tame your sweet tooth, the odds are stacked against you in the market place. That's because of a lab-engineered "bliss point" which is "a precise amount of sugar and fat and salt that will send consumers over the moon." See *Salt, Sugar, Fat: How the Food Giants Hooked Us* in Resources.

Given a choice between water sweetened with saccharin and intravenous cocaine, 94% of the lab rats opted for the sweet water, found this the <u>2007 French study</u>[7] *Intense Sweetness Surpasses Cocaine Rewards* by Avena et al. This is how packaged food and drink manufacturers use sugar to hook and condition us consumers like Pavlov's dogs.

Impaired Mouth Style vs. Proactive Healthcare

Your mouth style is how you use your mouth to open or shut the door on opportunistic infections and killer diseases. Beyond your immunity, each sugar hit harms you in many ways, be it fungal toes, wrinkled face, or senile brain. "Alzheimer's" disease was first recognized in 1910 by German psychiatrist Alois Alzheimer. It's now a household word and the most expensive medical condition to live with.

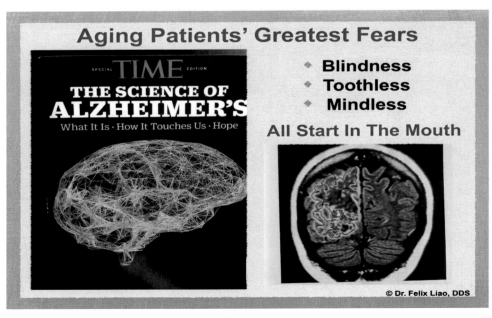

Figure 55

I once asked my dental patients: "What are your greatest fears in old age?" The top answers: loss of eyesight, teeth, and mind. Here's a proactive path: You can stop all three by becoming a smarter owner-operator of your mouth. My Rx: Avoid excess sugar and fix your Impaired Mouth.

Impaired Mouth Style (high sugar and processed foods) and Impaired Mouth Structure together add up to obesity, sleep apnea, teeth grinding, high blood pressure, erectile dysfunction, PMS, anxiety, fatigue, cancer, and COVID severity. In my opinion, all cardiovascular and metabolic diseases forming "foundational conditions" in COVID deaths can be traced to Impaired Mouth Style and Impaired Mouth Structure with choked airway. Talk to your doctor and AMD about how to best control your susceptibility.

Your Gut, Microbiome, and Immunity

Do you, or someone you know, have high blood pressure? Again, the mouth is the source. "The intestine is the largest bacterial ecosystem and immune response organ of the human body," reports a 2022 study[8] by Zhang et al. It links gut microbiome to hypertension associated with obstructive sleep apnea. "Intervention with probiotics, prebiotics, or postbiotics in animal models ... restored blood pressure to normal."

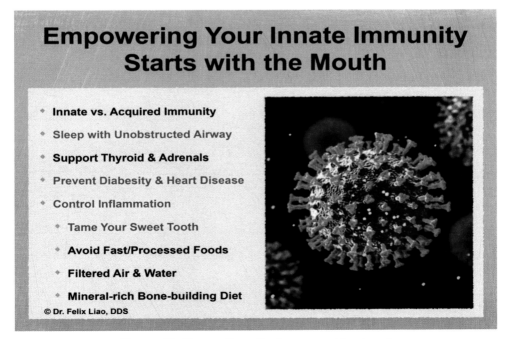

Figure 56. *More on the evils of processed foods and added sugar in Licensed To Thrive, chapters 5–10.*

Translated: What you eat either fuels or retards your immunity and high blood pressure.

So does what you go to sleep with: a wide-open or choked airway. A structurally sound mouth supports deep sleep, which in turn strengthens your ability to fight infections and illness. Conversely, an Impaired Mouth collapses airway, disrupts sleep, and deflates your immune resilience.

Snoring and Impaired Mouth: Two Peas in the Same Pod

Nasal breathing offers important filtering and immune protection against respiratory infections. Mouth breathing lets pollutants and microbes march right down your throat.

As Figure 57 shows, your nasal passage is a tunnel through your maxilla from nostrils to soft palate. This tunnel has a bony wall which communicates with several air chambers extending into the forehead and maxilla called sinuses. A soft tissue core warms, humidifies, filters, and immunizes the incoming air. The spaces between the soft tissues and bony wall are oxygen corridors. The less stuffy your nose and the wider your maxilla, the more air goes into your body.

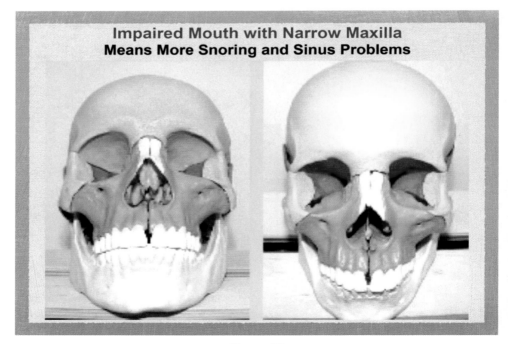

Figure 57

Snoring, a leading feature of Impaired Mouth Syndrome, is mouth breathing during sleep. This is often due to nasal tunnel blockage from:

- Narrow nasal tunnel from narrow maxilla.
- Congestion inside nasal tunnel from pollens, pollutants, dust mites, mold.
- Leaky Gut: reaction to foods and additives/preservatives/colors/chemicals.
- High stress, low downtime and poor sleep common in modern life.

Chapped, dry, peeling lips and parched tongue are signs of habitual mouth breathing, which also comes with weak lips (think sagging upper arm). Pink lips seen in healthy kids means vitality, while purple-ish or blue-ish lips at any age signal low oxygen and high risk. See your AMD or a myofunctional therapist for evaluation and for evaluation and treatment.

Nitric Oxide and Nasal Breathing

Nitric oxide relaxes the lungs to relieve breathing resistance, as Figure 58 shows, and opens blood vessels to lower high blood pressure. Nitric oxide is also the desired end product from taking erectile dysfunction pills. Your body makes nitric oxide naturally from nasal breathing.

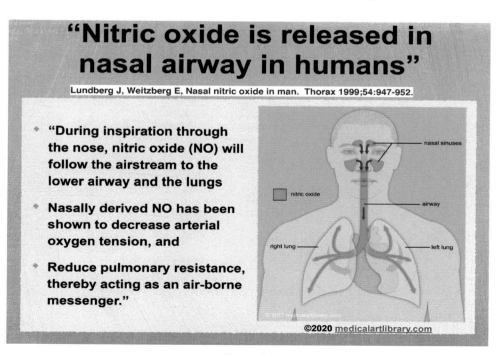

Figure 58

A deficient maxilla comes with a high and narrow palate and therefore a more cramped nasal passage. If you are susceptible to stuffy nose, snoring, sinus infections, colds and fatigue, you may have an undiagnosed Impaired Mouth.

WholeHealth Solution for Snoring

Snoring can be treated with an oral appliance to widen the "3-foot Cage", or an advanced painless laser to slim the "6-foot Tiger", or both.

Widening the palate with an epigenetic oral appliance also widens the nasal tunnel, since the floor of the nose is also the roof of the palate. This can improve nasal breathing and raise nitric oxide's beneficial effects on breathing and circulation.

FJ came as a new patient with CPAP intolerance for sleep apnea and erectile dysfunction. Both were fixed with the WholeHealth solution combining epigenetic oral appliance, bone-building diet, and myofunctional therapy. You can read FJ's case study in chapter 19 of *Licensed To Thrive*, or watch his comments by clicking *Follow Case Progress* in Resources.

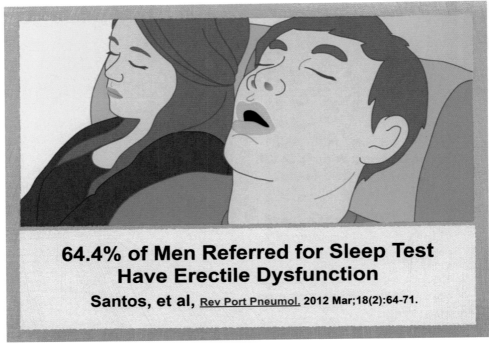

64.4% of Men Referred for Sleep Test Have Erectile Dysfunction

Santos, et al, Rev Port Pneumol. 2012 Mar;18(2):64-71.

Figure 59. *Consult an AMD to evaluate Impaired Mouth and choked airway as oral contributions to snoring, erectile dysfunction, and more.*

Before going to bed, I recommend snorers to check and unblock stuffy nose with Buteyko breathing exercise #1. See Resources. Your AMD can also provide referrals and suggest other resources. And always watch what you eat.

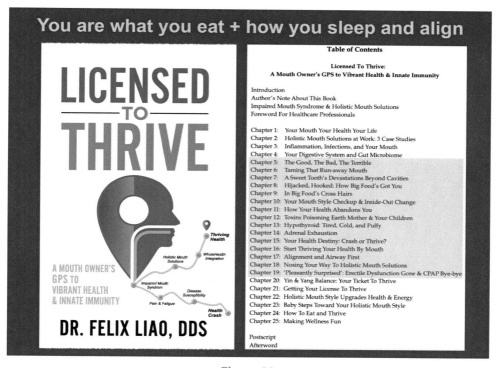

Figure 60

Painless Laser Treatment of Snoring

For faster relief from snoring, ask your AMD about painless laser treatment to tone and firm up your soft palate and tongue. It is a non-surgical and painless quick fix to reduce snoring while impaired Mouth style (eating and drinking against health) and impaired mouth structure are addressed over time.

Laser treatment applied to tongue and throat "may prove to be beneficial in non-surgical management of sleep apnea, especially the CPAP intolerant individuals," reported this 2015 pilot study[9].

Said pilot study has been confirmed in further research, including this 2018 report[10] which found "51-79% snoring [noise] reduction in non-smokers and non-obese individuals at 12 months after 4 laser treatments."

Eat to Thrive: A Vital Personal Wellness Skill

When you are stressed, hungry or tired, what's your go-to comfort food? Eating healthy in this era of ultra-processed foods (addictive chips and flavored and caffeinated drinks) is a vital personal wellness skill more crucial than brushing and flossing, in my opinion.

That roast chicken with two sides delivered to your door today is a far cry nutritionally compared to the same 50 years ago made in your grandma's kitchen. That's because our environment is far more toxic and our foods are increasingly tampered with. Please look at the trash generated by a takeout or delivered meal. I highly recommend these essential readings if you care about what you eat:

- *The Dental Diet* by Dr. Steven Lin. His book is a definitive guide on what to eat for your jaw and natural health in the 21st century.

- *Blood Sugar Solution* by Dr. Mark Hyman, MD, is an ultra-healthy program for losing weight, preventing disease, and feeling great.

If reading is not your thing, checkout the *Cook2Thrive* program in Resources by Chef Franklin to answer Dr. Lin's points in Figure 61.

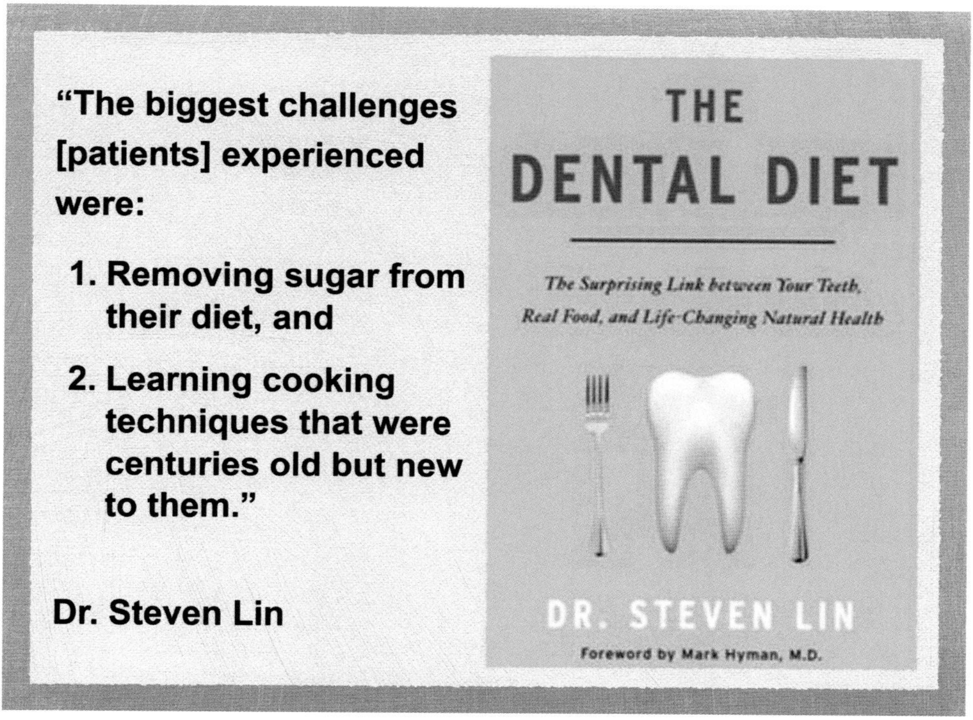

"The biggest challenges [patients] experienced were:

1. Removing sugar from their diet, and

2. Learning cooking techniques that were centuries old but new to them."

Dr. Steven Lin

THE
DENTAL DIET

The Surprising Link between Your Teeth, Real Food, and Life-Changing Natural Health

DR. STEVEN LIN

Foreword by Mark Hyman, M.D.

Figure 61

Cook2Thrive

Seventy percent of your immune system resides in the gut, as mentioned in this 2021 publication[11]. Did you know how to cook or eat healthy when you started to work and live independently? Nagging pain, chronic fatigue, and degenerative diseases start to show up 10-20 years later if TV commercials and pop-up ads regularly drive your food choices.

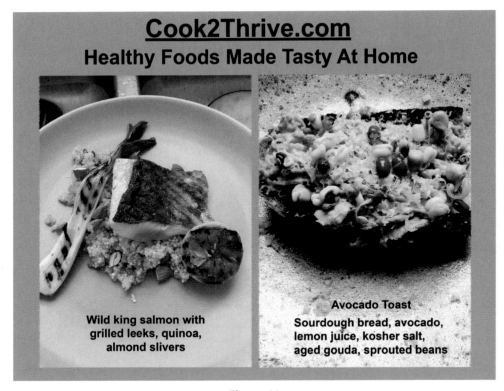

Figure 62

One hundred percent of your gut health hinges on how you operate your mouth. Learning to make healthy food tasty and fresh at home is a vital wellness skill to acquire, especially if you need to regrow your deficient maxilla and choked airway. See *Cook2Thrive* in Resources.

Conclusions:

- A structurally Impaired Mouth is more susceptible to snoring, sinus troubles, and cold and flus.

- Your Mouth Style is how you use your mouth to open or shut the door to opportunistic infections and degenerative diseases.

- Snoring is rooted in narrow maxilla, leaky gut and wrong eating. Knowing how to eat, improving lip strength and tone, and sleeping without airway obstruction add up to foundational solutions.

- The smartest way to stop suffering and start thriving is to:
  - learn to make fresh whole foods tasty in your own kitchen, and
  - have an Impaired Mouth evaluation by an Airway Mouth Doctor.

CHAPTER 6
STOP HURTING AND START THRIVING
See Your AMD About Your Airway and Mouth

You can take off your high heels or necktie when you go to bed, but you are stuck with your Impaired Mouth and choked airway when you go to sleep. Sleeping with an Impaired mouth brings on fatigue, and living with it piles on pain. Seeing an Airway Mouth Doctor or a trained non-dentist Airway Mouth Consultant can be helpful.

The mouth is where resuscitation takes place. Why wait until your life depends on going to the ER or ICU? With professional guidance and personal effort, you can stop hurting and start thriving at home and in your own bed.

Top of the Totem Pole

The mouth's place is the top of the healthcare totem pole, as Figure 63 shows. Dr. Chek's Totem Pole Hierarchy of Survival Reflexes independently agrees with my point: Fixing Mouth structure and Mouth Style are first-line treatments. Your mouth is the first place to look into if you have nagging pain and chronic fatigue. The next case is an example.

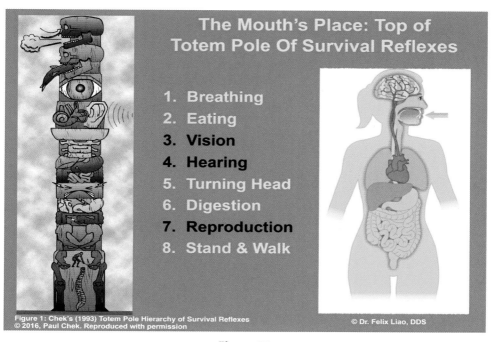

The Mouth's Place: Top of Totem Pole Of Survival Reflexes

1. Breathing
2. Eating
3. Vision
4. Hearing
5. Turning Head
6. Digestion
7. Reproduction
8. Stand & Walk

Figure 1: Chek's (1993) Totem Pole Hierarchy of Survival Reflexes
© 2016, Paul Chek. Reproduced with permission

© Dr. Felix Liao, DDS

Figure 63

Hope for All, Even Dental Amputees

QA came looking for an alternative to jaw surgery. That's after having four new adult teeth pulled and spaces closed with braces. Then four wisdom teeth were extracted, which left her with 24 teeth instead of the full complement of 32, and a far smaller space for her tongue between her now shorter and narrower jaws.

She was waking up 3–4 times every night and feeling tired in the morning 5–6 days a week. During sleep, she was grinding down her straight white teeth, causing her gums to recede. Her dentists had no answer for her since she had super-clean teeth with no cavities.

Figure 64 shows QA's signs and symptoms. Her tongue has been trapped inside a smaller "cage" ever since her dental amputations. So what's the way out?

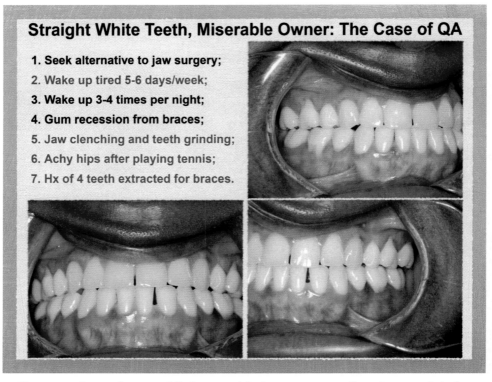

Straight White Teeth, Miserable Owner: The Case of QA

1. Seek alternative to jaw surgery;
2. Wake up tired 5-6 days/week;
3. Wake up 3-4 times per night;
4. Gum recession from braces;
5. Jaw clenching and teeth grinding;
6. Achy hips after playing tennis;
7. Hx of 4 teeth extracted for braces.

*Figure 64. Spaces between QA's front teeth before treatment reflect the struggle by her "Six-Foot Tiger Tongue" inside her "Two-Foot Cage" after her 8-teeth dental amputation. **Right** images: Gum recessions in her molars were present before starting oral appliance treatment.*

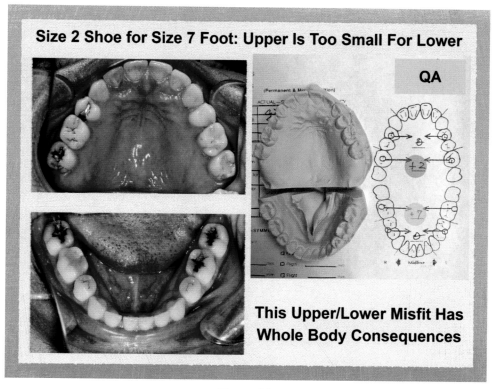

Figure 65

One key to break free from chronic pain fatigue is to regrow that "2-foot cage" into a more suitable habitat for the tongue. Slides 65–67 show the WholeHealth awareness and the diagnostics needed to solve such cases. Analysis of QA's Impaired Mouth revealed:

- Maxilla (upper jaw) was too small for mandible to fit in, as the numbers in the red and blue circles in Figure 65 show. This is a classic finding in pain and fatigue cases.

- Misfit between her maxilla and mandible contributed to her neck kink and hip pain, as shown in Figure 66.

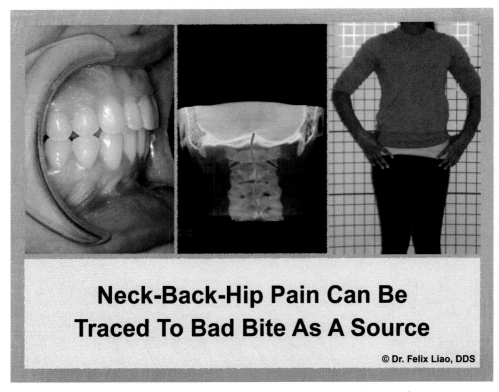

Figure 66. *QA's hands are on her pain zones after playing tennis.*

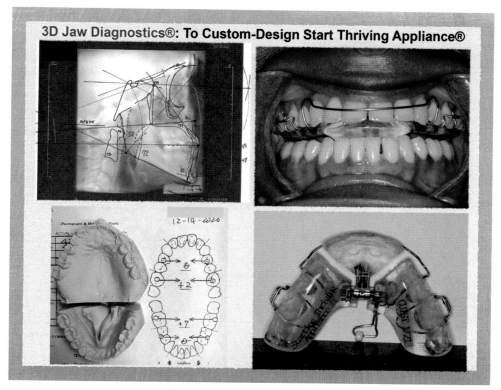

Figure 67. *3D Jaw Diagnostics® reveals Impaired Mouth and drives appliance design. Lower right image shows the amount of jaw growth in four months of treatment.*

Based on her 3D Jaw Diagnostics shown in Figure 67, a Start Thriving Appliance was made for her upper arch only. Her oral appliance was paired with a bone-building diet emphasizing homemade bone broth and fresh green smoothies, as shown in chapter 23 of *Licensed To Thrive*.

The results in QA's own handwriting are seen in Figure 68: "No longer waking up tired, no longer wake up with sore jaw, sleeping through the night, and no more hip pain after tennis."

This is how an Airway Mouth Doctor (AMD) who's trained in all the above and more can help fix chronic pain, fatigue, and raise life quality naturally without medication or surgery.

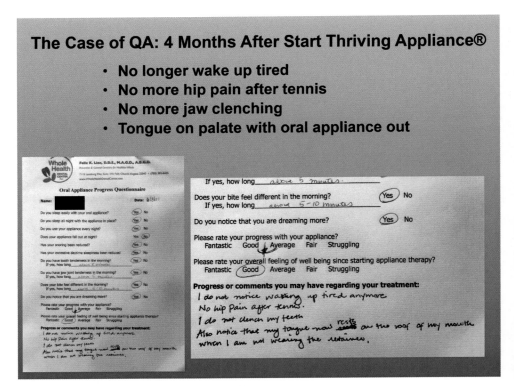

Figure 68

Take-Aways from QA's Case

- Airway relates to fatigue, and alignment relates to pain, and both have a huge oral contribution.

- More conservative and proactive solutions are now available.

- Recognizing Impaired Mouth is the first step to root out your pain and fatigue.

- Even in dental amputation cases, nearly all impaired Mouth symptoms can be improved with a correctly designed oral appliance and strong patient compliance.

Whether you have 32, 28, or 24 teeth, a trained AMD can help turn your Impaired Mouth into a Holistic Mouth to support Alignment, Breathing, and Sleep so you can enjoy life again.

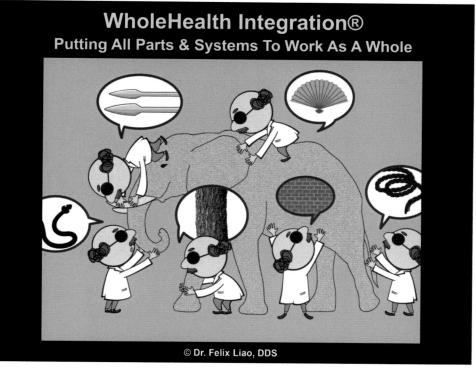

Figure 69. *The care of health starts with the mouth's role in airway, alignment, and eating, as* **Figure 63** *shows.*

SUMMARY

Relaunching your vitality starts with stopping chronic pain with mouth-body alignment and restoring deep sleep with a wide-open airway. Critical as the mouth is, shouldn't you have a mouth doctor well-versed in airway and alignment? That's why Impaired Mouth diagnosis has been missing. That's also why a new breed of dentist is sorely needed to upgrade whole body health.

Remember Dr. R's incisive comment at the end of chapter 1: "Patients cannot possibly know about Impaired Mouth if their doctors don't." This invites all dentists, doctors, and indeed all healthcare professionals to consider this question: "What else does this patient in front of me require besides my expertise?" See Cross-Training Summit in References.

Remember also SK's advice at the end of chapter 2: "I had to learn to trust that the healing comes from me." To the owner-operator of your mouth, it's time to take charge of your overall health and natural wellness by mouth. A trained AMD and/or AMC can be the Wise Wizard in your hero's journey to conquer pain, fatigue, and other symptoms of Impaired Mouth Syndrome.

Impaired Mouth Evaluation: The Key to Relaunch Your Vitality

An Airway Mouth Doctor (AMD) is a dentist with additional training after dental school to:

- Diagnose Impaired Mouth Syndrome to connect your symptoms to your mouth.

- Provide treatment to correct your impaired mouth structure and give guidance to improve your eating style.

- Coordinate WholeHealth team work to put your body's vital systems back in working order, as needed.

An AMD is not a formal graduate degree in dentistry. An AMD is a family dentist with the necessary WholeHealth knowledge and new skill set acquired after dental school to do the above in team work with other healthcare professionals as needed.

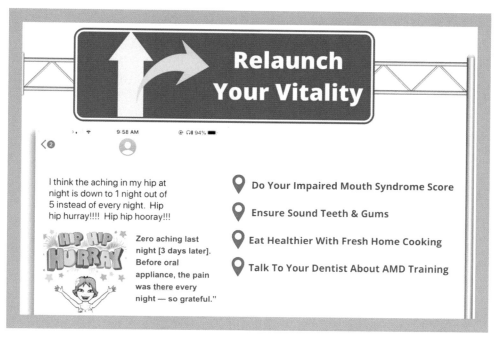

Figure 70

Finding & Seeing an AMD

This is your next step — the earlier the better:

- If your dentist is already trained as an AMD, you are in great hands.

- If not, you may need to nudge your dentist to get AMD Training so you can get your Impaired Mouth Syndrome treated in your current dental office. See Resources.

- If none of the above works and you cannot wait, please see Resources for a referral or an online consultation.

Finally, relaunching your vitality is within the reach of everyone with sound and sufficient natural teeth, regardless of age, with an AMD's help. Thank you for helping spread the word on this new possibility.

I wish you and yours thriving health.

RESOURCES

The following is intentionally kept short to stay focused. For a more complete list of references, please see bibliographies in the recommended books below.

1. **AMD Training for Dentists:** Text/call 800-969-8035

2. **Follow Case Progress:** https://bit.ly/RelaunchYourVitality

3. **Airway Mouth Consultant Training for Non-dentist Healthcare Professionals:** Please email info@HolisticMouthSolutions.com

4. **Telemedicine consultation for a fee:** Email request to info@WholeHealthDentalCenter.com

5. **Cook2Thrive**[12] with Chef Franklin: Thrive Your Health Through Your Kitchen for busy working professionals

6. **Cross-Training Summit for non-dentist healthcare professionals to cross-refer and collaborate with AMDs on WholeHealth integration:** info@HolisticMouthSolutions.com

Books by Dr. Liao on Impaired Mouth Syndrome & Whole-Health:

1. **Six-Foot Tiger, Three-Foot Cage:** *Take Charge of Your Health by Taking Charge of Your Mouth*

2. **Early Sirens:** *Critical Health Warnings & Holistic Mouth Solutions for Snoring, Teeth Grinding, Jaw Clicking, Chronic Pain, Fatigue, and More*

3. **Licensed To Thrive**[13]: *A Mouth Owner's GPS to Vibrant Health & Innate Immunity*

4. **Your Child's Best Face**[14]: *How to Nurture Top Health & Natural Glow*

On Healthier Diet, Weaning, and Sleep Breathing:

1. **Academy of Orofacial Myofunctional Therapy**[15]: Its members and AMDs combine to form leading-edge expertise in physical therapy for the tongue, lips, cheek, and swallowing muscles

2. **Salt, Sugar, Fat**[16]: *How The Food Giants Hooked Us*, by Michael Moss

3. **The Dental Diet**[17] by Dr. Steven Lin

4. **The Blood Sugar Solution**[18]: *The UltraHealthy Program for Losing Weight, Preventing Disease, and Feeling Great Now!* By Mark Hyman, MD

5. **The Weston A. Price Foundation**[19]: *Wise Traditions Diet*

6. **Nurtured Bones Newsletter**[20]: *Concise and consistently excellent tips on bone health*

7. **Sleep, Interrupted**[21]: *A physician reveals the #1 reason why so many of us are sick and tired*, by Steven Y. Park, MD

8. **Sleep with Buteyko**[22]: *Stop Snoring, Sleep Apnea and Insomnia* by Patrick McKeown

9. **Breath**[23]: *The New Science of a Lost Art*, by James Nestor

10. **Stop the Snore**[24]: *Dental Solutions for Healthy Sleep*, by Gene Sambataro, DDS

CONTACT THE AUTHOR

Emails:
Dentists, Doctors, Healthcare Professionals: DrFelixLiao@gmail.com
Patients & Readers: DrFelix@HolisticMouthSolutions.com

Websites:
For healthcare professionals: www.HolisticMouthSolutions.com
For patients seeking consultation: www.WholeHealthDentalCenter.com

Facebook:
For healthcare professionals: www.facebook.com/HolisticMouthSolutions
For patients seeking consultation: www.facebook.com/wholehealthdentalcenter

Instagram:
www.instagram.com/6_foot_tiger

LinkedIn:
www.linkedin.com/company/HolisticMouthSolutions

Vimeo:
www.vimeo.com/wholehealthcsiminibooks

REFERENCES

1. Molin, L.D. *A User Guide to: Using the SUDS Scale to Measure the Intensity of Feelings.* Available Online: https://inneractions.com.au/downloads/SUDS_Scale-Intensity_of_Feelings_Measure.pdf. Accessed November 14, 2022.

2. Liao, F. *Six-Foot Tiger, Three-Foot Cage: Take Charge of Your Health by Taking Charge of Your Mouth.* Crescendo Publishing LLC; 2017. Kindle Edition Available on Amazon: https://www.amazon.com/Six-Foot-Tiger-Three-Foot-Cage-Charge.

3. Liao, F. *Early Sirens: Critical Health Warnings & Holistic Mouth Solutions for Snoring, Teeth Grinding, Jaw Clicking, Chronic Pain, Fatigue, and More.* Crescendo Publishing LLC; 2017. Kindle Edition Available on Amazon: https://www.amazon.com/Early-Sirens-Critical-Warnings-Solutions-ebook/dp/B0762S8G9B.

4. Cenzato, N., Nobili, A., & Maspero, C. (2021). Prevalence of Dental Malocclusions in Different Geographical Areas: Scoping Review. *Dentistry journal*, 9(10), 117. https://doi.org/10.3390/dj9100117.

5. Blue Zones. https://www.bluezones.com/recipes/food-guidelines. *Food Guidelines.* Accessed November 14, 2022.

6. Albert Sanchez, J. L. Reeser, H. S. Lau, P. Y. Yahiku, R. E. Willard, P. J. McMillan, S. Y. Cho, A. R. Magie, U. D. Register, Role of sugars in human neutrophilic phagocytosis, *The American Journal of Clinical Nutrition*, Volume 26, Issue 11, November 1973, Pages 1180–1184, https://doi.org/10.1093/ajcn/26.11.1180.

7. Lenoir, M., Serre, F., Cantin, L., & Ahmed, S. H. (2007). Intense sweetness surpasses cocaine reward. *PloS one*, 2(8), e698. https://doi.org/10.1371/journal.pone.0000698.

8. Zhang, L., Ko, C. Y., & Zeng, Y. M. (2022). Immunoregulatory Effect of Short-Chain Fatty Acids from Gut Microbiota on Obstructive Sleep Apnea-Associated Hypertension. *Nature and science of sleep*, 14, 393–405. https://doi.org/10.2147/NSS.S354742.

9. 2015 pilot study: https://www.oatext.com/pdf/DOCR-1-113.pdf. Lee C.Y. & Lee C.C. (2015). Evaluation of a non-ablative Er: YAG laser procedure to increase the oropharyngeal airway volume: A pilot study. *Dent Oral Craniofacial Res.* 2015;1:56–9. https://doi.org/10.15761/DOCR.1000113.

10. Laser & Health Academy. http://www.laserandhealth.com. Accessed November 14, 2022.

11. Wiertsema, S. P., van Bergenhenegouwen, J., Garssen, J., & Knippels, L. M. J.; 2021. The Interplay between the Gut Microbiome and the Immune System in the Context of Infectious Diseases throughout Life and the Role of Nutrition in Optimizing Treatment Strategies. *Nutrients*, 13(3), 886. https://doi.org/10.3390/nu13030886.

12. Cook2Thrive: https://www.cook2thrive.com. Accessed November 14, 2022.

13. Liao, F. *Licensed To Thrive.* Crescendo Publishing LLC; 2020. Kindle Edition Available on Amazon: https://www.amazon.com/Licensed-Thrive-Owners-Vibrant-Immunity-ebook/dp/B08R93GNB4/ref=sr_1_1?crid=2RS4XK6VJGFWN&keywords=licensed+to+thrive+-book&qid=1641055620&s=books&sprefix=licensed+to+thrive+book,stripbooks,89&sr=1-1.

14. Liao, F. *Your Child's Best Face.* Holistic Mouth Solutions Media; 1st edition; 2022. Kindle Edition Available on Amazon: https://www.amazon.com/dp/B0BK9WS7MX.

15. Academy of Orofacial Myofunctional Therapy. https://www.aomtinfo.org. Accessed November 14, 2022.

16. Moss, M. *Salt, Sugar, Fat.* Random House Trade Paperbacks; Reprint edition; 2014. Kindle Edition Available on Amazon: https://www.amazon.com/Salt-Sugar-Fat-Giants-Hooked/dp/0812982193.

17. Lin, S. *The Dental Diet.* Hay House, Inc.; Illustrated edition; 2018. Kindle Edition Available on Amazon: https://www.amazon.com/Dental-Diet-Surprising-between-Life-Changing/dp/1401953174.

18. Hyman, M. *The Blood Sugar Solution.* Little, Brown Spark; 1st edition; 2012. Kindle Edition Available on Amazon: https://www.amazon.com/Blood-Sugar-Solution-UltraHealthy-Preventing-ebook/dp/B004QX07AK/ref=sr_1_9?keywords=Mark+Hyman&qid=1641056868&s=books&sr=1-9.

19. The Weston A. Price Foundation. https://www.westonaprice.org. *About the Weston A. Price Foundation.* Accessed November 14, 2022.

20. Nurtured Bones. https://www.nurturedbones.com. Accessed November 14, 2022.

21. Park, Y.P. *Sleep, Interrupted.* Jodev Press, LLC; 1st edition; 2008. Kindle Edition Available on Amazon: https://www.amazon.com/Sleep-Interrupted-Steven-Park-M-D-ebook/dp/B002R5B2GM.

22. McKeown, P. *Sleep with Buteyko: Stop Snoring, Sleep Apnoea and Insomnia, Suitable for Children and Adults.* Buteyko Books Loughwell, Moycullen, Co. Galway; 2017. Kindle Edition Available on Amazon: https://www.amazon.com/Sleep-Buteyko-Insomnia-Suitable-Children-ebook/dp/B08L3S85V3/ref=sr_1_3?crid=2UZVE22MQXDIH&keywords=patrick+mckeown+books&qid=1641639276&s=digital-text&sprefix=Patrick+Mck,digital-text,91&sr=1-3.

23. Nestor, J. *Breath: The New Science of a Lost Art.* Riverhead Books; Later Printing edition; 2020. Kindle Edition Available on Amazon: https://www.amazon.com/Breath-New-Science-Lost-Art/dp/B082FPZC4H/ref=sr_1_1?gclid=Cj0KCQjwxlOXBhCrARIsAL1QFCY0cDLCZVwfIVUKttaVjo8gSlsCI5l6hTIFrNAItqDaREYkb-GYpdg0aAieCEALw_wcB&hvadid=558517680951&hvdev=c&hvlocphy=9008138&hvnetw=g&hvqmt=e&hvrand=13137207998831598939&hvtargid=kwd-913763104543&hydadcr=22533_10353821&keywords=breathe+nestor&qid=1668549929&s=books&sr=1-1.

24. Sambatro, G. *Stop the Snore: Dental Solutions for Healthy Sleep.* Advantage Media Group; 1st edition; 2017. Kindle Edition Available on Amazon: https://www.amazon.com/Stop-Snore-Dental-Solutions-Healthy/dp/1599328658.

Made in the USA
Middletown, DE
15 October 2023

40862000R00055